Pilates Without Tears

The 5-Step No Pain No Strain Strategy to Move and Feel Great

Jeannie Di Bon

London, United Kingdom
www.createpilates.com
E: create@createpilates.com
T: +44 208 879 9840

For information about special discounts for bulk purchases, please contact 10-10-10 Publishing at 1-888-504-6257

ISBN-13: 978-1523694174

PUBLISHED BY:
10-10-10 PUBLISHING
MARKHAM, ON
CANADA

Contents

This book is dedicated to my husband Ilario for his unending support, encouragement and passion. I am truly grateful to him.

Acknowledgements

I wish to acknowledge all those that have made this book possible:

- My husband for continually supporting and telling me I could.
- My children for inspiring me.
- My clients for being my greatest teachers.
- My fantastic team at Create Pilates, London.
- The amazing educators and mentors I have had the privilege to work with, both in the United Kingdom and the United States.
- The Pilates and Yoga communities for the extraordinary wealth of knowledge they have made available to practitioners. I have been honoured to be exposed to it and have developed my own interpretation of functional and effective movement.
- Vanda Scaravelli, who sadly I did not meet, but whose words of wisdom have inspired me so much in writing this book.
- Justin Ward for creating beautiful photographs and his patience!

About the Author

Jeannie Di Bon has been teaching Pilates since 2008. She has trained with internationally renowned organizations – Body Control Pilates, Polestar Pilates and The Pilates Method Alliance – and world-class educators in the United Kingdom, Europe and the United States.

She is the owner and managing director of her successful Pilates Studio in London, UK – Create Pilates. She writes regularly in her own Blog at www.createpilates.com.

Jeannie's specialism is rehabilitation, back-care and sports performance working extensively with runners, tennis players, golfers and skiers. She works closely with leading medical professionals on a regular basis.

She is a firm believer in examining many schools of thought and aspects of movement to cultivate programs uniquely tailored to each individual, enabling them to feel strong, flexible and great.

Praise for Jeannie Di Bon

Through working with Jeannie, I was able to complete all my training and the London Marathon without injury. The strength I built up during my weekly sessions helped to power me along the 26 mile route and across the line! Thank you to Jeannie.
Rosemary Thorpe, Client

Until I had the opportunity to work with Jeannie, I had no idea Pilates could be like this. Her method is very effective: it has enabled me to understand my body and resolve pain issues by adopting a very holistic approach.
Natasha De Grunwald, Bowen Practitioner

The benefits of a consistent Pilates practice are so far reaching. Having been troubled for many years from post knee replacement pain, I now enjoy pain free walking. Not only have I become stronger, I have shaped up too! The threat of a second knee surgery no longer exists thanks to the exercise guidance I have received. My medical team have been amazed! I sleep better now and feel invigorated for life.
Vanita Patel, Client

Foreword

There are many exercise books on the market today and we are well informed on the need and benefits to move and exercise more. This first book by Jeannie, Pilates Without Tears, came to my attention for a number of reasons. First the title caught my eye: from what I know of Pilates, this title really stood out and I was curious to learn what it meant. I have found out that this book is not the usual, traditional exercise manual – it is a lifestyle game changer.

Jeannie's many years of teaching experience and deep passion for educating and empowering people shines through on every page. She explores movement within a broad scientific and psychological context and uses Pilates as the foundation of her method. She makes Pilates accessible for everyone – from those who are in pain or suffering stress related illnesses to performance athletes – and teaches them how to change their whole relationship with movement. Throughout the whole book I have felt that Jeannie is speaking with the reader personally, and is supporting their journey of discovery and transformation.

I would recommend this book for anyone looking to understand the deeper underpinnings of why we move and how we do it, beyond simply showing how to make it look good. It is a very well thought out and explained journey that I wholeheartedly invite you to undertake.

Raymond Aaron
New York Times Best-Selling Author

Why This Book? My Story.

Pilates Without Tears - I am sure there are many picking up this book and thinking what a strange name for a book. You may be saying to yourself "Pilates does not bring me tears; I love Pilates. Pilates makes me feel strong, fit and toned. I am more flexible than ever before." Absolutely! We read in the media every day how Pilates is used by so many types of individuals in a versatile way; it is the recommended exercise by healthcare and medical professionals for back pain, it is used for the management of chronic pain, world class sports teams use it as part of their training programmes to build strength and help prevent injury. People as young as 7 are now taking weekly classes to combat the onset of postural problems. Pilates has no age limit - people up to their 90s are practising it as a part of a regular routine to keep agile, flexible and mobile. People's lives have literally been transformed by the regular practice of Pilates and the freedom and relief from pain they have found. I personally do not believe there is any other movement and exercise method that can touch so many people. There are no tears after Pilates. But what if you have been in pain doing exercise? What if you have been searching for a method that you can use to change how you approach movement? Maybe you have developed fear of movement because if often causes pain. What if you've always pushed hard all your life, pushing your body to the limits physically and emotionally? What if you could change your thoughts and approach to movement? What if there was a different way that allowed your body to start to move naturally, the way it was designed to, without force and discomfort and yet you felt stronger, more connected and freer? There are many Pilates exercise books on the market - this is not an exercise book. It will not take you through advanced poses and repertoire, as it is not designed to compete in that market. This is written and designed to be an integrated approach that goes beyond the performance of an exercise, to challenge you to delve deeper beyond the exercise.

What do I mean by this? What is Pilates Without Tears? I have been teaching since 2008. Over the years, I have worked with many types of clients, from elite athletes to those suffering from chronic pain, to those wanting to enjoy the benefits of regular Pilates. I noticed an underlying trend in the majority of the clients, which I wanted to examine and explore through the method I have now come to name the Integral Movement Method. There were not literal tears of course (although there was a certain amount of frustration and anger with their own bodies sometimes) but this book is an attempt to put into words the remarkable changes I have seen in my own clients. The trend I noticed, which came both from clients totally new to Pilates or clients who had been practising Pilates somewhere else, is best described as a 'tension led' movement leading to a disconnection throughout the whole system. I had felt in my own body that the body is deeply connected - one thing is going to influence and impact everything else. What I was seeing, however, was a disconnection with the body, disconnection with the mind, disconnection with what was going on. It was almost as though the body was individual parts. Arms, legs, spine, feet. A knee fold was an exercise to lift the leg - which it is to a certain extent, but what else goes on there? What are the implications of that movement for the person? A ribcage closure was an exercise to raise the arms - but just the arms. I saw no integration of the arms into the body. I saw no integration of the breath with the use of the arms. By that I was not looking for cueing the inhale and the exhale, but I wanted to see the breath help create and facilitate the movement at every level. It simply was not there. Sometimes clients would demonstrate advanced exercises but I could not remove the fact that I saw tension and strain in many cases. There was a sense of force rather than grace. Exercises were often performed to "do" the exercise regardless. Clients would often say "Well I've been doing this exercise, but it hurts here." When I looked at the moving body as an integrated global system, not at individual body parts, I could just see the tension in the body. No wonder it was hurting in some cases. I found that if I retaught the exercise with my Integral Movement Method, the pain and tension could be eliminated. The movements changed dramatically to my eye, and the clients felt the change instantly.

So, I began to experiment. I tried different cues, different ideas, I explored and studied different movement practices branching out from the Pilates arena. I began to mix all these elements together. I began to ask questions to the clients such as "What are you thinking of when this happens?", "What do you feel when you do this?", "How did you get to where you are now in this exercise?" First, clients were thrown by being asked how they felt; what did I mean by this? I sometimes thought they had never been asked how they felt before.

Through the Integral Movement Method I want to bring that connection back to the client's awareness - because it is already there within the body. We've lost our awareness. My method is a way to help clients reconnect, to find their natural movement and enjoy the natural elasticity and connectivity within. Movement becomes effortless, which means less energy consumed and a greater vitality.

I believe Pilates is so much more than exercise. It is not about looking pretty on the mat - it has to be done with ease and fluid integration. We have to look at the implications of any movement on the body as a whole, and start to take away that unnecessary tension and stress which sadly is often created when trying to "do" Pilates or indeed other exercises - rather than really observing what the body needs and craves. There are often metaphorical tears of frustration, pain, stress and restrictions. I wanted to create a method where clients did not have Pilates with tears! Why should it hurt? It shouldn't. Why should it be a massive effort as opposed to a journey of exploration and inquisition?

The Integral Movement Method and my way of teaching have evolved over the years and have been influenced by many schools of thought and movement practices, including Pilates, yoga, in-depth anatomy and biomechanical training. I was particularly drawn to the work of Vanda Scaravelli, an Italian yoga teacher who studied with Iyengar. Her book *Awakening the Spine* is a beautiful piece of work which resonated with how I had been teaching for many years. I began to question why I had never seen this approach in Pilates. There is a method of Scaravelli-inspired yoga; I guess I would call my work Scaravelli-inspired Pilates.

Like many people, I first discovered Pilates after being recommended to try it by a physiotherapist. I had been seeing the physio for a number of months for shoulder and neck pain. I had recently had two children in a relatively short space of time and I had little time or energy to take care of my body. A niggling shoulder developed into a chronic issue. One day he told me "You are hanging off your joints, you have no stability or core." I had no idea what he was talking about - this was how I was and I had no body awareness of what my posture and habits were inflicting on my body. He handed me a Pilates book and told me to take it home and read it. What a revelation that book was! It had a list of symptoms that could be caused by poor posture - headaches, neck ache, shoulder pain, lower back pain. I was just running through that list ticking them all off! I was hooked, and booked myself into my first Pilates class the very next day. I loved everything about it - so much that I knew very early on that this was a practice I wanted to delve deeper into and share and teach with others. The journey began then to become a Pilates and movement teacher. I love what I do and I love sharing my passion with my clients.

This book is a culmination of my experiences, thoughts and interactions with my clients, and is written for my clients and people like them - maybe like you too. It is for those who have been in pain, including chronic low back pain, those returning from long-term illness or stress-related illness or symptoms. It is also for those high achievers who have been used to pushing hard to achieve what they want - maybe you still want to be a high achiever, but are looking to manage the stress that tends to go with that more effectively. And, it is for anyone who wants to move and feel great by learning a different strategy of listening to your body. The no pain, no strain approach, plus a fit, toned body without the bulk. Long and lean!

My clients have often requested that I put something on audio or a book so that they can carry our work with them all the time. For many years I laughed this off but the requests kept coming. I am honoured that so many would wish to learn more, and am grateful for this opportunity to share my thoughts. So here it is - my first book written and published. I thank my clients for being so vocal and encouraging me to put pen to paper.

This book will share with you the foundations behind my way of working, and will explain the Integral Movement Method. I will share with you the 5-step plan that I use with every client with amazing results that are achievable at home with practice, patience and persistence. It also serves as a practical guide on how to apply this method to your life every day.

The book is structured to allow you to follow the method as I do. Chapter One explores the implications of breath - breath permeates everywhere and everything. There is no better place to begin. Chapter Two brings us to the floor - the role of the feet in allowing the body to free up tension. This is where we spend most of our time - the understanding of their role is crucial. Chapter Three takes us straight into the concept of the global system I have described above. This book would be incomplete without a mention of the 'core' - Chapter Four challenges some beliefs about this concept. Chapters Five and Six begin to delve deeper into the premise of removing these 'tension-led' movement patterns and encouraging you to discover the easiest way to move. Chapter Seven prepares your mind for the Integral Movement Method - the focus, the motivation and the awareness are uncovered. We are completing the book with the 5-step strategy in Chapter Eight, followed by detailed foundation exercises in Chapter Nine which you can follow and practise at home.

I truly hope it serves its purpose for people being able to benefit from working in a different way, to discover a new approach to movement, to looking at their minds and bodies with a heightened focus and sense of awareness. It is deliberately not a technical manual or an anatomy book - I wanted to make it easy to read, follow and, most of all, apply. The book itself is like a journey, an unravelling of what is currently in place in your body and your mind, and it is a reprogramming of our habits, our gestures, our way of moving. If you can proceed through each chapter in order, each chapter will take you deeper into your understanding of your body and will make more sense.

You will notice the book poses many questions to you as you progress through the chapters. This is deliberate - I always question my clients. Why? Not because I am looking for a perfect answer, not because I am judging them at all, but for them to bring awareness to what has taken place. To challenge their views of the world, their bodies, their reactions to their bodies. I seek to increase their sense of awareness because with awareness we can make a change. Without we are just doing! I celebrate when a client says "I feel different," "I feel strange or weird." Yes! Celebrate the difference because in that very moment your body has taken a step out of the norm. Or, what your body perceives as the norm - even if it is high stress and pain.

A new journey lies ahead. Enjoy the journey!

Jeannie Di Bon

CHAPTER ONE
BREATH IS EVERYTHING

Breath is everything - without it we wouldn't be around for very long! So what do I mean by this?

Breath is the very essence of movement. It is so integrated into the ability of the body to move freely that it can never be overlooked. To dismiss the breath as an integral part of any practice means you are missing out a major element and connection with your body. Practising and embedding this into your body will allow you to access this not just in an exercise class, but every day.

Later in this chapter, we will examine some breathing exercises to practice, but for now some very simple anatomy.

The thing that amazes clients so much is that the majority of your lung tissue is located in the back of your body, not the front. I think we assume the lungs are in front because of our breathing practices today and our inability to breathe into the back of the body. I use the word inability loosely because this is something that can be re-learnt - it is not a given. Our lifestyles today are very much in front of us - we sit at computers, we drive, we watch television and reach for the remote or smartphone. For the majority of our daily life, we are pretty sedentary. The media is full of the new line "sitting is the new smoking" highlighting the dangers of this passive approach to life. An article in The Huffington Post (September 2014) highlights how researchers now claim prolonged sitting causes serious illnesses such as cancer, heart disease and type II diabetes. We are no longer required to move dynamically - everything is at our finger tips, automated. Our focus has become the front of the body - over time our breathing patterns will adapt to suit this.

You may be already having an internal dialogue with yourself thinking it cannot change the fact that you have an office based job ; this is just how it is. The fantastic news is that it is changeable. Keep reading!

KEY MESSAGE NO 1 - NOTHING IS STATIC IN THE BODY, EVERYTHING IS CHANGEABLE

There are 3 breathing patterns I refer to with clients - Accessory or Clavicular Breathing, Lateral or Thoracic Breathing, and Belly Breathing. Let's try them out now in this explorative exercise. I do this with every client and it is a really effective way to bringing awareness to our current breathing habits - good and not so good. You can do this lying on your back or seated in a chair. If you are happy to, close your eyes. Spend one minute minimum on each pattern.

KEY MESSAGE NO 2 - THERE IS NO RIGHT OR WRONG. DO NOT HAVE ANY EXPECTATIONS OF DOING IT RIGHT

EXERCISE - KNOW YOUR BREATH

Accessory or Clavicular Breathing: place your hands lightly on your sternum / breastbone. Notice the hands resting there. Breathe into the area where you feel the weight of your hands.

What happens there? Is this a new sensation? Is it comfortable, normal? Do you feel the sternum rise and fall with each breath?

Where is the movement happening for you? Do your shoulders rise on the inhale? Do you notice any tension around the neck?

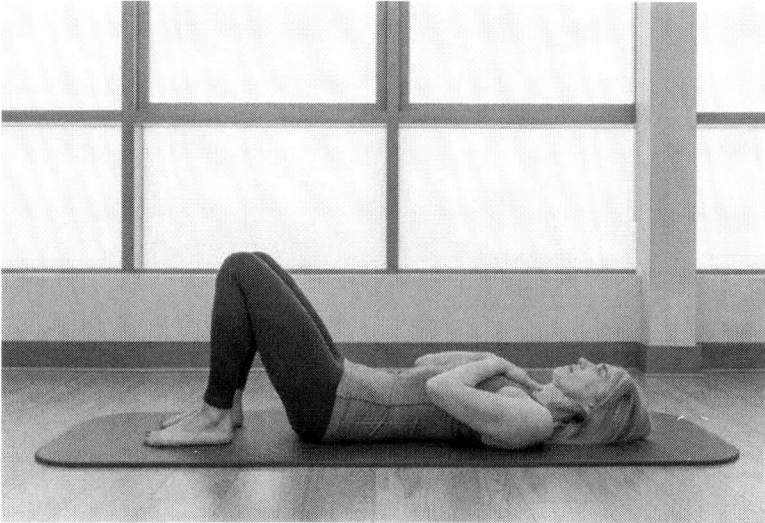

Fig 1

Lateral or Thoracic Breathing: place your hands around your lower ribcage. If possible, try to place the four fingers at the front of your body and the thumb behind so that you are holding as much of the ribcage as possible.

Breathe into your hands. What happens? How does it feel? Easy? Challenging? Frustrating? Where does your breath go in this very moment? Do you feel the ribcage move? Do the ribs feel sticky or stuck? Does one rib move more than the other side? Where is the movement?

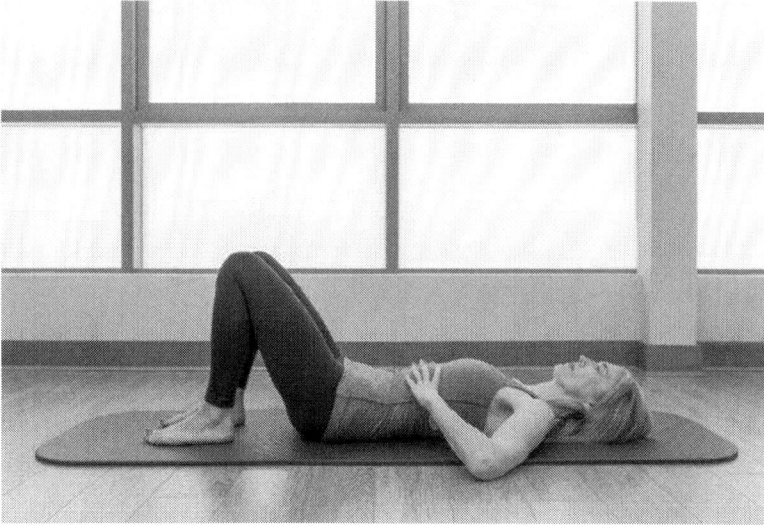

Fig 2

Belly Breathing: place your thumbs in line with your belly button and your fingers pointing downwards towards your lower abdomen. Breathe down into your hands. How does that make you feel? Is it a normal pattern for you? Do you feel the belly rising and falling? Can you allow the belly to soften as you exhale? Does the belly rise as you inhale? Does your spine or pelvis move as you perform this pattern?

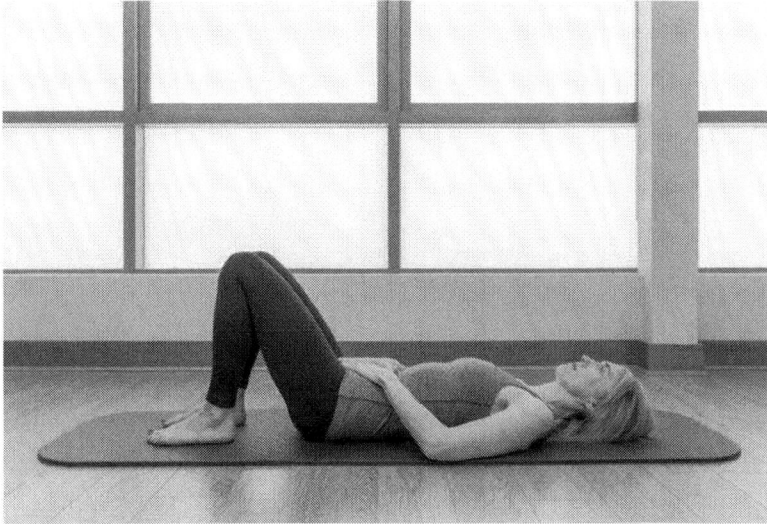

Fig 3

When you have completed all three areas with at least one minute on each, rest your hands by your side.

POST EXERCISE QUESTIONS

- Which pattern felt most comfortable?
- Which one felt normal; is it your pattern?
- Which one felt new, challenging?
- Did any cause a sense of impatience, frustration?
- What did you observe or learn about your body doing this exercise?

Visit my website www.pilateswithouttears.com to claim your free bonus of an audio version of this exercise. You can continue to practice the exercise with some guidance from me.

You may have identified some new information about your breath. None of these are incorrect but you may have discovered you favoured one or maybe two particular patterns. Individually they may start to inhibit the body. This will not just be in terms of movement freedom, but everyday life.

Accessory breathing tends to be a shallow breath, often seen when your body is stressed. It is also the response after physical activity - the body is attempting to bring air into the body quickly. If you have ever run very fast and stop because you are out of breath, maybe bending forward, hands on knees - this will be automatic accessory breathing as you try to catch your breath. As a long-term breathing strategy, this is not ideal. We are not fully accessing the lung capacity, which over time will diminish without use. We barely inhale past the collarbone. Accessory breathing muscles are muscles that have an assisting role in breath, but it should not be their primary role. Muscles of the neck, upper chest and back can start to be involved with too much emphasis. This can cause stress and tension around the head, neck and shoulders.

I personally was a rib-gripper, an addict of over-trained lateral breathing. I was taught the importance of lateral breathing in my original Pilates training, but not in the context of complementing this pattern with the other patterns. The result of years of rib-gripping was the inability to let my belly expand when I inhaled. I was, after all, a Pilates teacher - shouldn't I always have a firm, toned belly?! And the inability to let my belly relax led to an overactive pelvic floor. If you are constantly gripping and using the abdominal muscles on a daily basis, you are going to be using your pelvic floor in an unnatural way. Even though it felt so wrong to let my belly relax initially, I now relish in the freedom it has given me.

We want to ensure we are using the diaphragm efficiently when we are breathing. With contraction of the diaphragm, the belly expands on inhale, rather than just the sternum or the chest. The diaphragm is a large dome-shaped muscle at the base of the lungs, and is the most efficient muscle for breathing. Yet, so many of us lose the ability to breathe correctly and use this muscle. Your abdominal muscles help move the diaphragm so these should naturally respond to your breath. They should not, therefore, be held or sucked in during the process of inhalation and exhalation as is so often cued in Pilates and exercise classes.

What we are seeking in a healthy breathing pattern that serves us well is a full body breath encompassing all 3 patterns together with the ability to access the lung tissue at the back of the body - 3 dimensional breathing. We need to be there with our breath too.

EXERCISE - OPEN YOUR LUNGS

Initially, this exercise will be easier if performed lying on your back, knees bent, feet flat on the floor. A minimum of 2 minutes will be required but you may find you want to stay longer. Please use a cushion to support your head if your neck feels any discomfort.

Rest one hand on your sternum and one on your belly. Notice the hands resting. Gently, without excessive force, try to inhale down into the belly, ribs and sternum in that order - like you were filling a cup with water. Feel the torso expanding with the air.

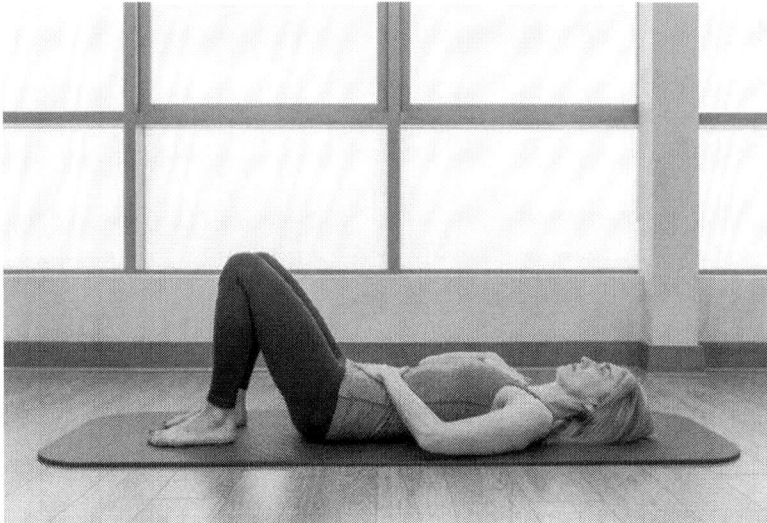

Fig 4

As you exhale, empty the belly first, then the ribs and finally the sternum - as though you were emptying a bath. Feel the air leave the body.

We start to bring the breathing together and full. Try this for a few rounds of breath. Try not to hurry or force the breath.

Now, at the same time, envisage drawing the breath into the back of your throat towards the base of your tongue. Try to imagine you are breathing without a nose. Maybe you have gills like a fish instead at the sides of your head. We begin the direct the breath to the back, not the front of the body. You may feel some pressure into the mat as your lungs expand back and down. This is normal. Allow the front body to be quieter as the air is spread between the front and the back body. Do not be disheartened if this feels strange or difficult. If you have been breathing into your front body for many years, the body needs to learn a new pattern. With regular practice, this will become the normal pattern. What is important is that we explored all 3 patterns and in doing so you discovered an area that could be improved for your better health.

POST EXERCISE QUESTIONS

- How did it feel?
- Was it a different experience than the first exercise?
- Where did you notice the breath go?
- Did the breath favour the front body?
- Did you notice one side of your body respond more quickly?
- What did you notice about the pace of the breath - did it change?
- How do you feel post exercise?

There will be further breathing exercises in Chapter Seven.

To develop awareness of your breath, continue to observe and practice this method. I would like, however, at this stage to introduce another layer of information. I call this first section the technicalities of breathing - the how to. This is important to master but we can go further into the body's response to your breath. This will be needed as we come to the exercises later in the book as it forms one of the foundations of the Integral Movement Method.

KEY MESSAGE NO 3 - IF I TAKE AWAY THE NEED TO DO, I CAN BE TRULY PRESENT

We rarely stop to think of our breath on a daily basis - we take on average 15-20 breaths per minute - that's a massive 20,000 a day (American Lung Association). To notice every single one would drive us crazy and leave little thought for anything else. But to spend time with our breath has enormous physical and emotional benefits. Physically, as we have just experienced in the exercise Open Your Lungs, if we retrain our breathing muscles, we can increase our lung capacity, we can massage the internal organs and expand the muscles that could otherwise be untouched by the breath. Your spine is lengthened and massaged by your breath. Your joints find space and freedom with breath. Muscles that may have been overworking 20,000 times a day can start to switch off a little.

What about the emotional connection of breath? We already spoke of accessory breathing tending to be a stress response. When someone feels ill or is inconsolable, we tell them to take a deep breath. There is clearly a connection with breath and emotion. Let us try to use our awareness of our breath to tune in deeper to our feelings, to connect deeper with our body. This awareness will be invaluable further into the book and your daily life.

EXERCISE - FIND SPACE WITH YOUR BREATH

Resume your position of lying supine with your knees bent, feet flat on the floor. You can rest your hands by your sides, palms facing up or down. Allow your eyes to close. Please use a cushion or folded towel to support your head if your neck is in any discomfort.

Begin the Open Your Lungs breathing practice as outlined in the previous exercise. Do not be hurried or in a rush to get somewhere. Notice the internal dialogue - the chit chat your brain is trying to have with you. Let it pass and return to your breath. The mind will become quieter in time. All you are doing right now is observing the breath - watching the inhale, watching the exhale. Notice it - no two breaths will ever be the same. Notice how the breath becomes slower and quieter. On your next inhale, could it have so little force that a person standing next to you could not hear you? "Receive the air in a passive detached way as though you were only an observer." (Scaravelli, Awakening the Spine).

All too often we feel we need to breathe - we take massive inhales through our nostrils. That action alone can cause muscle tension around the head, neck and shoulders. Our strategy in this book - The Integral Movement Method - is to find a new way of moving that eliminates stress and tension whenever we can. Given that we breathe 20,000 times a day, the breath is going to have implications on this. How can it not? This is why I spend a good deal of time with my clients on their breath. It is at the heart of all movement you try to do, be it a Pilates class, or running a marathon, or pushing a shopping trolley.

As your inhale quietens, notice the mind has too. Notice the exhale and what it gives you. As your breath leaves the body, can you start to feel the weightiness of your own body? Imagine you are lying on a foam mattress and every out-breath causes you to sink further into the mattress. You sink so deep that when you stand there will be an imprint on the mattress of your body, your spine. Can you see the shape of your bones? What will that imprint look like? Would one side of the body be heavier? Would there be a deeper imprint in some areas? Do you see a balance of your imprint - the head and pelvis weighing the same? What does the alignment look like - did you lie straight on the mattress? Are there rotations or twists that you sense?

Allow your body to soften - the bones, the muscles, the tissue. The weight of your body sinks to the back. You feel your organs weighted down underneath you. As the body softens, it lengthens and widens. You are creating space, spinal elongation, and joint space with your breath. Your imprint has changed shape again. (Key Message No 1 - nothing is static). Even in lying, your body is not still; it will change and morph as the breath moves it.

Spend time enjoying the quiet of the inhale and the softening of the exhale. This is true rest. No demands on your time, nobody asking anything of you. You are a quiet observer of your body.

POST EXERCISE QUESTIONS

- How did it feel to breathe with full awareness of what was happening?
- What new awareness did you have of your body?
- Did you notice any resistance in your body to let go?
- How busy was the mind? Did it become easier?
- How did you feel after the exercise and for some time afterwards?
- If you had a picture now of your imprint, what would it tell you?

The exercise we have just completed allowed us to experience the role gravity has to play in our bodies and our movement potential. By allowing your body to sink and soften, you began to work with gravity rather than fighting it. This is a huge step - congratulations. This leads us on to the following chapter, where we explore working with gravity in greater depth.

You can visit www.pilateswithouttears.com to download your own free audio copy of this exercise - Find Space With Your Breath.

CHAPTER TWO
FEET FROM THE GROUND UP

How often do you think about your feet on a daily basis? We decide what shoes to wear to work, put the shoes on, and off we go for the day, probably not paying our feet much attention - unless of course they hurt. Maybe our shoes rubbed and we got a blister, or our feet were hot and swollen on a summer's day. Other than that, I am guessing feet are not a top priority. They certainly were not for me, until I started to really study their anatomy, structure and critical role they play in relation to what happens further up the body. Then feet started to get really interesting and they became a bit of an obsession for me. I was fascinated by what I had learnt and seen, and started to share this information with my clients in their Pilates classes and one-to-one sessions. The changes were profound and amazing. I started to see people moving in a totally different way. My clients probably never go a single lesson with me without hearing a reference to the feet. They are crucial to our body's well- being and health. I am not a biomechanics specialist; this section is not designed to compete with the many excellent books on the market about the foot, gait analysis and the intrinsic working of the foot. I use my knowledge and study of the foot and apply its functionality and role within an integrated body to Pilates and movement. I believe the foot is often overlooked in the Pilates arena, and I want to draw attention to this.

Here's why - let's begin with a brief and simple anatomy of the foot.

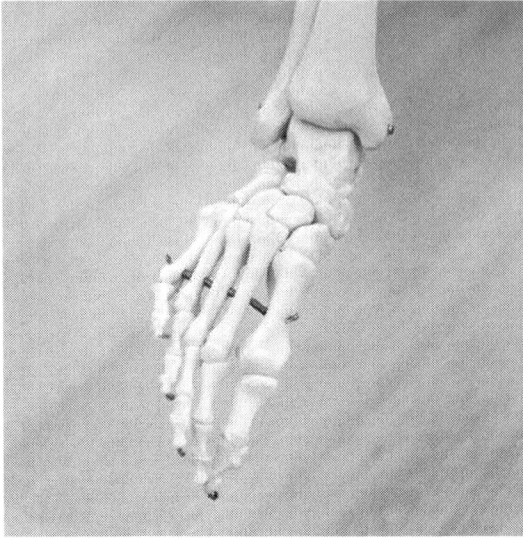

Fig 5

Your foot has 33 joints and 26 bones - that's just one, so multiply that by two. The spine also has 33 joints and 34 bones. That is an equal number of moving surfaces in both your foot and your spine. That is a massive amount of potential movement in a foot that gets placed in a shoe and forgotten about all day. It is really like wearing a straight-jacket on your spine. Imagine how stiff and uncomfortable it would be to bind up your spine for just one day. Gary Ward, author of *What The Foot*, questions "Isn't the impact of movement in each of your feet therefore equally as important as movement in your spine?" I have to agree, and I spend a lot of time explaining to my clients that what goes on at the feet will have a huge impact on everything else. Hence, I have put this chapter right at the front of the book. That's how important they are to me - and you, hopefully by the end of this chapter.

Do you ever walk barefoot? At home and work I always walk barefoot and try to do so (where it is safe and free from potential harmful objects) outside too. When I do wear shoes, I try to vary the style every day and not to wear the same pair two days in a row. The reason I do this is to give the muscles and joints in my feet variety and challenge. If I were to wear the same shoes every day, 12 hours a day and then go to bed, my feet would not have had much of a workout. Imagine it this way - what would happen if you put your hands in mittens for 12 hours a day? How functional and responsive would they be? And yet, this is what we do to our feet. When I walk barefoot, my feet are forced to encounter uneven surfaces and different sensations, and they start to wake up. Most of our sensory receptors are in our hands and feet, but we cover and suffocate 50% of these for most of our day. Think of all that information your brain is missing out on receiving. A sensory receptor is a sensory nerve ending that responds to a stimulus inside or outside the body.

When I look at the foot with its 26 bones, 33 joints, muscles that run up to the lower limb and knee and a large portion of sensory receptors, I cannot help but think how can this not be of importance? The position of the feet, the degree of pronation (flat footed) will influence the spine. If one foot is more pronated than the other - which is very likely - what impact will that have? Why not try it now - stand up and allow one foot to role inwards so that most of the weight is on your inner side of your foot. How does that feel? Balanced? Do you feel tension more on one side of the body? Do you notice how you have to twist your legs and pelvis just to stand upright?

I believe the feet are meant to be flexible enough to move and respond to the ground underneath, and stable enough to support the weight above it. Of course our ancestors walked barefoot, climbed trees, jumped and ran for miles every day and likely had this natural organisation in their structure. Due to our

modern lifestyles, we have lost touch with our feet and the huge
benefit they can have on removing pain, stress and tension in
your body. Let's start to wake them up and use them how they
are designed to be used.

Feet come in all shapes and sizes, and degrees of mobility. There
are rigid feet with little mobility or very flexible floppy feet with
no stability, and more than likely a combination of both. I have
yet to find a perfect foot that looks like the anatomy books, but
all feet have potential and ability to change. This includes flat or
over-pronated feet.

So where do we start to find a stable yet flexible, responsive foot?
When I meet with a new client, I always start from the ground
up. I ask them to stand barefoot and I stare at them for a good
length of time. I examine the feet and how they are presenting
themselves. I trace the patterns from the feet up the body and
start to build a picture of what might be going on in this
particular body's organisation. Where is the alignment, what
patterns do I see, how do the patterns of the feet follow the pain
the client might be experiencing in their body? And I ask the
client a lot of questions.

The challenge is for us to rediscover our feet - as discussed, most
of us have lost touch with them. This is where Pilates studio
equipment such as the Reformer, Chair and Trapeze Table really
come into play, but much can be achieved without access to
these machines.

EXERCISE - DISCOVER YOUR SOLE

Assume a standing position with bare feet - in whatever feels
comfortable and pain free. Remember Key Message No 2 - there
is no right or wrong. At this stage I want you to be pain free -

we will work on alignment later. This exercise will take a minimum of 5 minutes.

Close your eyes, if you are happy to. If you have a balance disorder, please keep your eyes open.

Notice how you feel, how you are standing, notice the thoughts coming in and out of your mind. Notice any tension in the feet, around the ankle or up the calf to the knee or lower back.

Send your attention down to your feet and observe them. How do they feel? What surface are you standing on? How does the surface feel under your feet? Where do you feel most of the weight in your feet? The front or the heels? Are you aware of your toes? Do they all touch the floor? Does one foot feel heavier than the other? Does one foot feel bigger?

Imagine you are now standing on wet sand at the beach. Can you allow the feet to sink into the sand? With every exhale, you sink deeper into the sand. Can you make a soft imprint in the sand? As you stand on the sand, the feet sink deeper and the imprint becomes wider and longer at the same time. Your base of support becomes larger.

When you step away from your imprint, imagine looking down at it. What does it look like? Is one imprint deeper than the other? One foot bigger than the other? Are the feet straight on or turned out?

Allow your eyes to open and stand quietly for a moment.

POST EXERCISE QUESTIONS

• Did you feel different at the end of the exercise?
• Did you notice any tension in your lower limb before the exercise and did this ebb away during the exercise?
• What did you observe about the weight falling through your body to your feet?
• What did your imprint tell you about how you might be holding your body?
• Did you notice your feet for maybe the first time in years?

There will be further exercises coming up in Chapter Three.

You can receive a free added bonus of this exercise with an audio download at www.pilateswithouttears.com.

As we start to practise this first foot awareness exercise, the brain starts to reawaken the neural pathway and pay more attention to the feet. We need to build this fundamental awareness into our bodies. I see the feet as very much being our foundations. They need to be solid and grounded. I often use the analogy of a tree with my clients; the feet are the roots of the tree that go way beyond the surface, they are drawn down into the ground by the pull of gravity. The roots reach out in many directions representing the stability and flexibility of the feet. Our legs and pelvis are the trunk also being drawn down towards the feet - there is a weightiness to them that allows the torso and arms to rest of them comfortably. From the pelvis up, there are the branches and leaves - the parts that move freely in the wind, with a lightness and grace. As Vanda Scaravelli stated "The spine moves simultaneously in two opposite directions." It is also referred to as opposition - movement in two directions at the same time.

What I am seeking, therefore, when working with my clients, once we have established some degree of awareness of the feet, is the ability to allow the foot to respond to its environment. When the foot responds and begins to work effectively, the branches above are required to do less. The spine feels security from its roots; it has to work less to hold the body up against the downward pull of gravity. We need to do less fighting with gravity and begin to work with it. "All movements we do against the flow of gravity are negative." (Scaravelli) Then we start to see real freedom in the spine. If you have ever stood on a wobble board or BOSU or such balance equipment, you will notice how insecure you initially feel, and the body assumes a rigidity to compensate for the lack of stability below. With practice, however, the feet respond and adapt to this unfamiliar feeling, and the body is able to find its centre and lose that rigidity.

EXERCISE - OPEN YOUR FOOT

This is a simple standing exercise to allow us to explore the foot and allow it to unravel. Begin standing with your bare feet beside each other. Lift one leg and place the heel of the foot in front of you as though you were taking a small step forward. From the heel, allow the foot to roll forward and down to the ground until the whole foot is on the floor. Allow the foot to roll, expand lengthways and widthways as it makes contact with the floor. Take a look at your foot and see if it changes shape as it makes contact.

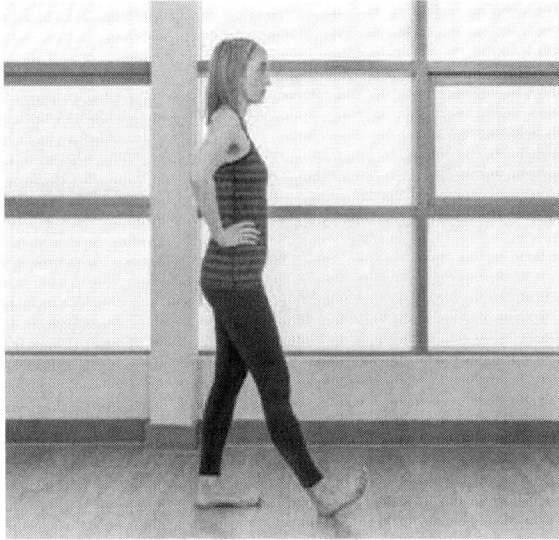

Fig 6

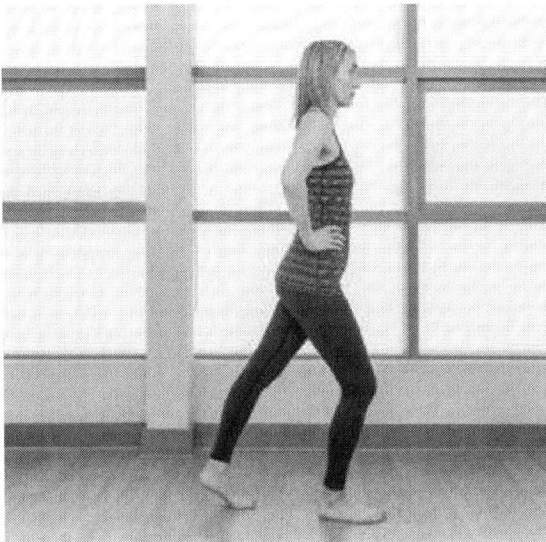

Fig 7

Allow the foot to meet with the floor softly, with awareness of each part of the sole touching the floor, and allow the foot to open up. It is similar to when you drop olive oil on a counter - it forms a blob of oil and then it expands. The oil becomes dispersed - this is what we want the foot to do - move in multiple directions.

Try the other foot.

POST EXERCISE QUESTIONS

- Did you notice a change in your foot?
- Did you notice the joints and bones move apart?
- Did you want to grip your toes?
- Did one foot respond differently to the other?
- Was there any pain, stiffness, tension in the foot or calf?

KEY MESSAGE NO 4 - IF MY FEET DO MORE, THE REST OF MY BODY CAN DO LESS = MORE EFFICIENCY, MORE ENERGY, GREAT NEWS!

A well-organised foot leads to a well-organised body. Awareness of the role of the feet is essential to reaping the benefits of the Integral Movement Method. Continue to explore, massage and mobilise your feet as we continue into Chapter Three - Your Body Is A Tent.

CHAPTER THREE
YOUR BODY IS A TENT

I know the saying is "my body is a temple" and it should be, with regards to the substances and food we put into our bodies - that's a whole other topic that is definitely worth exploring, but for the purposes of this book and the Integral Movement Method, your body is now a tent.

I always use this analogy with my clients as it is an image everyone can relate to. Even if you have never put up a tent, you certainly know what one looks like and the concept of how to put it up. So hopefully it's an easy idea to grasp.

When you put up a tent it is important to have the right amount of tension in all the guide ropes. The central pole frame needs to be firmly grounded and the ropes come from this centre out into space. If I manage to establish my tent structure with balance - the same amount of tension around the whole tent - my tent is going to be able to withstand the wind and rain. If, however, one or two of my ropes are slightly weaker or they haven't been given the same amount of tension as the others, I have a potential problem. I could be ok initially with little wind but, day after day, that structure will be put under more strain. The tent may start to sag or droop on one side. If there is a storm or strong gusts of wind, my tent could collapse.

This is how I want you to start looking at your body. This is not an anatomy book where we will go through individual muscles and parts - we want to start viewing the body as a whole unit. We have explored the feet as they are crucial to your tent's

31

stability and durability, but that's as far as we go now in terms of individual structures. Your feet are part of your whole and your whole is affected by your feet. It's a dynamic relationship that is constantly changing, adjusting and settling.

Your body is an integrated unit. Remember Chapter One where we first explored the breath and how it could change the body's relationship with gravity. We were not yet moving - think of the possibilities when we do!

During one of my anatomy training courses, the class was introduced to this exercise. I love sharing this explorative exercise with clients - we often have a lightbulb moment after this.

EXERCISE - WHAT MOVES ME

Assume a standing position. If you have a mirror, it is great to observe what happens. Take hold of the bottom edge of your top and start to scrunch up the material on one side. Notice the change in the tension in the material. Can you feel the fabric being pulled taut across your body? Imagine if you continued to pull and scrunch the material - I would imagine your top would soon become misshapen, or maybe develop a small tear.

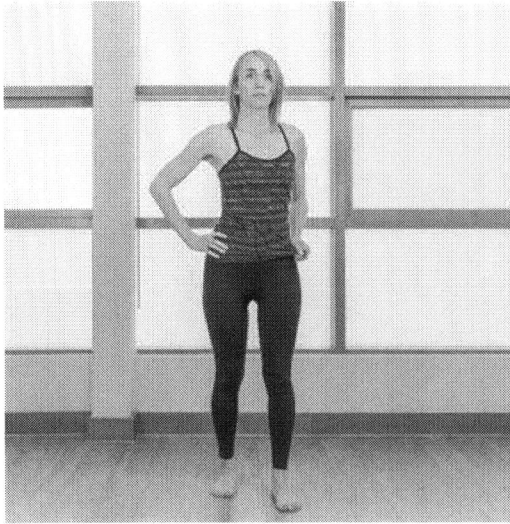

Fig 8

POST EXERCISE QUESTIONS

- How did you feel as the material became tighter?
- How did your skin feel underneath your top?
- What would it feel like to walk around like this for an hour, a day, a week? Would it drive you mad?
- Would you feel a restriction after a week?

Now, this was just from a force from the top. If you were wearing a full head to toe body suit, and you repeated the exercise, the force would be coming from the top and bottom - a pull in more than one direction.

Imagine trying that for a week, a month, or a year.

Guess what - that's what we do. We just cannot see it, we certainly don't do it deliberately as in the exercise, but we can normally feel it. Some muscle tightness, restriction or pain - that's a sign that your tent is out of balance, one of your guide ropes has been pulled too tightly or maybe it has become too loose and unstable. But just as in the case of your body suit, the internal structure inside your body is being pulled in different directions in an unbalanced way.

So what is this internal structure?

The internal structure is connective tissue - fascia. Fascia, according to leading expert Robert Schliep, is the "soft tissue component of the connective tissue system that permeates the human body." In other words it envelops everything! It connects muscles with each other and the skeleton. The fascia provides a wrapping for the organs, the vessels and the nervous system. It is a bit like the skin around a sausage. It has an amazing role - it is sensitive to the lightest of touch, it communicates around the body, it tenses up when we feel threatened and it expands when we are under the right conditions. "It is the most important organ for proprioception." (Robert Schliep) Proprioception is the body's ability to sense movement within joints. It allows us to know where our body parts are in space, and the role of fascia to communicate this information is critical. Furthermore, fascia is also capable of storing and releasing kinetic energy just like an elastic spring.

So sensitive, intelligent, responsive! This is a powerful organ. How can we start to work with it to harness this amazing power? In exercise or life, if we try to force our bodies to move in a way that communicates a threat to the system, such as an aggressive and forced stretching, your body may fight you back. For example, have you ever tried to stretch your hamstrings? Did it hurt at the back of the legs? If you are a regular hamstring stretcher, how often do you stretch your hamstrings? Do you ever notice a change from one day to the next? In other words, are the hamstrings always tight no matter how much stretching you do? You may need a different approach if you answered yes. Our body often resists when we force a stretch that it is not ready to accept. We have to ask why the hamstring muscles are so tight or loose. Yes, muscles can hurt just as much if they are stretched too long and have become stringy and ineffective. Maybe it is not the fault of the poor hamstrings that keep getting forced to stretch more. Maybe we sit down for 90% of our day and the hamstrings are just not functioning effectively anymore. They are weakened by lack of inactivity. With an unwanted force, the body can feel threatened and the fascia contracts, the muscles shorten and we defeat our objective of trying to stretch. Try approaching this with a different mindset of a gentle softening into the movement. Use of breath will assist in allowing the body to release (as per Chapter One) and the action of softening will free up space and freedom in the body. The body will be happier to accept this change rather than being forced into a position that it is not ready to take. We will try this exercise out together in Chapter Six.

If we return to the analogy of our body suit, if I have tension and restriction somewhere in my body, the fascia is going to be pulling in many different directions. It will not be a linear pulling. I had the honour of attending a couple of human dissections on cadaver in London. It was an absolute privilege to be able to explore the body, the layers of tissue, muscle, organs. There is more on this experience on my blog at http://www.createpilates.com/blog if you would like to read the full piece. The key take-away was that the body is a huge spiral - the bones are cylindrical and the muscles wrap themselves around the body in overlapping spirals. There are NO straight muscles. The muscles lay over each other and slide on top of each other - a sliding matrix of spirals. There is no start or finish

- the muscles run into each other. The body certainly does not look like the pictures we see in anatomy books - with perfect drawings of individual muscles all perfectly cut and presented.

KEY MESSAGE NO 5 - THERE ARE NO STRAIGHT LINES OR HARD EDGES IN THE BODY. EVERTHING SPIRALS AND WE DO NOT FUNCTION IN STRAIGHT LINES.

As the body is a complex network of connective tissue, how can we isolate a movement in Pilates or any other exercise? How can we talk of an exercise being a "glute" exercise or an "abdominal" exercise? How can it be just a hamstring stretch? It just cannot be - whatever you do is going to have implications and consequences for the rest of the body, and that includes the bits we can see on the outside and the bits we cannot see on the inside. My pet hate is the use of cues such as "push your bottom into the air and squeeze your glutes as hard as you can" or similar such strange cues. This is my personal rant and it drives me crazy. Apologies if I get passionate about this and I will elaborate more why in Chapter Four, but I really feel it is a disservice to the body to communicate to it like this. It is designed to operate as a whole - why does the fitness industry insist on cutting it up into little pieces? If we want to strengthen our glutes, great! I am totally in agreement with that, as most of us have sleepy glutes from too much sitting and not enough activity, but there are other, more intelligent ways to talk to your body. And your body will thank you for it.

A well-organised body will give you strength, power, flexibility and stability. Let's take a global view of the body - you are not just a glute or a rectus abdominus or a bicep. Why treat your body like that?

KEY MESSAGE NO 6 - MY BODY REALLY IS A TENT AND NOT INDIVIDUAL PARTS. I AM WHOLE.

CHAPTER FOUR
SO WHERE'S MY CORE AND HOW CAN I MAKE IT STRONGER?

This is a tricky subject which has been argued about and written about for many years. The term "core stability" first arrived in the 1990s and was largely derived from studies carried out to look at trunk control in patients with low back pain. Influences from Pilates have promoted several assumptions about core stability training, such as weak abdominal muscles lead to back pain, strengthening the abdominal muscles will reduce back pain and a strong core will prevent injury (Lederman, The Myth of Core Stability). This resulted in a whole fitness industry explosion of core stability training in gyms and classes calling for bracing of the trunk and 'tummy tucking' and 'navel to spine hollowing.'

Many people talked of the importance of the Transverse Abdominus (TrA) which does play a role in the trunk stabilisation, but in synergy with every other muscle of the abdominal wall and beyond (Lederman). Lederman also reports that despite the call for strength training of these core muscles to minimise back pain and reduce injury, it seems that the trunk muscles do not need a great deal of force to stabilise the spine. During standing and walking the trunk muscles are at minimal activation. So, that means we don't need to go around bracing and squeezing to get a result! Thank goodness for that!

Lederman states "It is doubtful that there exists a 'core' group of trunk muscles that operates independently of all other trunk muscles during daily or sport activities." In other words, everything is connected! (see Chapter Three) Plus, "To specifically activate the core muscles during functional movement the individual would have to override natural patterns of trunk muscle activation," meaning we would be exaggerating and overworking our bodies unnecessarily by squeezing and pushing and forcing! We don't need to do this because our bodies know how to move anyway. Another yippee from me!

One final point - "muscle by muscle activation does not exist," because it's all connected. Remember, your body is a tent! We can certainly focus on an area, pay attention to that area and build sensation around it - as we did in our feet earlier - but we are never working that one area alone.

What I find this most interesting from Lederman's study is that, in terms of abdominal muscle strength training, he found abdominal hollowing was the most ineffective form and did not increase stability. Wow! Bracing did improve stability, but at the cost of spinal compression! Wow again! So why do people continue to do it and want to feel the pain?!

I personally have never spoken to my clients about squeezing muscles or bracing or hollowing. It never felt correct or a normal activity. When a dog runs for a stick in the park, I have never seen it stop, suck in his abdominals, brace himself and then attempt to move. He just moves, and his body knows what to do and when. I never saw the reasoning behind messing around with the natural programming in the body, confusing it and teaching it an unnatural way of moving. Clients often come to see me for the primary reason of "strengthening their core" and they pat their stomachs as they say this. We have been conditioned and led to believe by the media that our core is our abdominals - the TrA and Pelvic Floor.

When I first started teaching, I took on a new client for one-to-one sessions who told me she wanted to do Pilates because she wanted a flat stomach and therefore wanted to do lots of curl-ups in every session. I went along with it out of inexperience and the desire to keep the client happy. I did what she thought she needed. Her stomach did not get flatter. I was disappointed and so was she.

This was many years ago. Today, with my greater practical experience and deeper knowledge of anatomy, I can confidently educate my clients that this approach simply will not work. As we discussed in the previous chapter, everything is connected. Working your abs by doing lots of curl-ups or sit-ups will not give you the body you desire. If I over-tighten the front of my body, shorten the muscles enough to maybe even give me an aesthetically pleasing six-pack, what is going on at the back of the body? Am I going to get a nagging lower back ache because the muscles have been pulled long to allow the front to shorten? Maybe. Am I going to get a hernia because of so much tension in my abdominal wall? All that crunching could eventually lead to something breaking through the wall. The abdominal area is essentially a water-filled sack. If you ever filled a balloon with water as a child and squeezed it, what happened? The pressure has to go somewhere. The water either gets pushed in opposite directions or the balloon explodes. I'm not so keen on that idea for my body!

Pilates today is a fantastic discipline in this regard - a well thought-out class should have the appropriate amount of flexion, extension, rotation and lateral flexion in it. It allows your body to experience all ranges of movement in balance. I always feel a little sad when I read comments on social media of people having attended a Pilates class and they comment "Don't think I will be able to walk tomorrow; my glutes hurt so much" or "Am really going to feel my abs tomorrow after that Pilates class."

Why? Why is this a good thing? Are we strengthening our 'core' by doing this? I'm not so sure. Are we creating a body out of balance? Are we doing potential harm? Don't even get me started on the ever-popular gym classes called legs, bums and tums!

I personally don't like the word "core", and try not to use it. But if I were to describe it, it is like an apple core. It runs through the whole centre of the body, with the softer fleshy pieces on the outside. The core, from my perspective, starts at the feet (see Chapter Two) and works its way up through the inside leg including inner thighs, pelvic floor, abdominals and spine, through to the roof of the mouth - where the spine meets the skull. If this is well-organised and accessed by the sensory mind, we start to feel many things - connection, strength, elongation, alignment, centring; there is an appropriate amount of tension in the body - I simply call it "good tension". We want tension in the body - without it we would look like a sack of potatoes. If I can arrange my body so that I have the correct amount of good tension, I have a core. In my opinion, that is how you access your 'core.' The core is not just muscular, it is sensory, and it goes deeper than the surface. It is a feeling, a way of being. With this tension, as we were discussing the abs earlier, the abs would know how to respond in relation to the rest of the body. They are not isolated, disconnected, trained to work alone but with fluid integration to the rest of the structure.

EXERCISE - FIND YOUR APPLE CORE

Let's revisit the exercise Open Your Foot from Chapter Two. Establish a standing posture where you have connected with your feet, your roots, and feel a weightiness from the pelvis down.

From this place, think of an apple core that runs through your centre. Begin the journey at the feet and get a sense of this apple core growing upwards through the legs. Do not hurry the breath - it is as though every out-breath draws the core a little further up the body. It is a sense of organic growth rather than just being there. It is intrinsic with the breath. Follow the journey. As it passes through the pelvic floor, abdominals and up through the deep spinal muscles, gain a sense of elongation and lightness. Follow it with eyes closed to the roof of the mouth, where its integration from the ground gives a place for the weight of the head to rest. Similar to a plate balancing trick.

From that strong apple core running through the centre, allow the periphery (arms, shoulders, outer edges) to fall, suspended from the core. Almost a sense of being draped over the core. There is no effort in holding your body up. Allow the body to settle into this place of quietness with an inner strength that comes from deep within your senses. Can you find a place here of no tension?

POST EXERCISE QUESTIONS

- Were you able to feel the growth through your centre?
- Did you lose connection at some point?
- How did you feel at the end? What words would you use to describe it?
- How would it feel to have this feeling every day?
- How integrated was your breath to achieve this sense in your body?
- Would it have been possible without breath awareness?

If you enjoyed this exercise and wish to try it with some audio, simply visit www.pilateswithouttears.com to claim your free bonus download of this exercise.

The fantastic news is that this feeling is achievable every day. In fact, it can become who you are, how you stand, how you move. Practiced with awareness and patience, we can have this sense of lightness and connection as our normal state. The Integral Movement Method is a way of moving that works to eliminate stress and tension from the body, allowing you to feel a sense of release and new-found freedom. My clients often say to me that they never knew they were holding tension until we work through the method to let it go. They are amazed at how they have been operating through life carrying this tension with them. That has become their habit through no fault of their own. The great news is that habits can be broken and new habits made. I totally understand where my clients are coming from because I too was one of those people. I remember an incident in my late twenties, before I had discovered Pilates. I was working in the City of London in a big accountancy firm. One evening I was washing up at the kitchen sink and I noticed that I was gripping my legs and my glutes. My shoulders were rigid as I went about my task of washing dishes. I stopped momentarily and observed this. I was so unaware and disconnected from my body that I did not even realise this was wrong. It had become my norm. It was who I was. I look back now and see how much wasted energy was in that person. It has been an absolute revelation to me to discover a body that can let go and yet become stronger. The less I try, the stronger I become. To me, this is a true 'core.'

This leads us on to our next chapter: No Pain, No Strain.

CHAPTER FIVE
NO PAIN, NO STRAIN

Our lives have become so demanding on our time. We have technology at our fingertips, which is a great innovation but it also means we cannot escape so easily. People can contact us anytime, anywhere and ask things from us. They make demands on us - emails, texts and social media. This, coupled with all our pre technology activities of running a home, looking after children, and working full time can lead to stress and a sense of being overwhelmed. We always feel like we should be DOING!

What this invariably leads to - I see it every day in the studio - is this continuation of the sense and need to be DOING! We need to do exercise as it is the right thing to be doing, we need to do Pilates because it is good for our bodies, we need to do more and keep doing more! Yes of course, everyone should be exercising - data from the World Cancer Research Fund (September 2015) states that a third of cancer cases in the UK alone could be prevented if people exercised more and ate healthily. But, can we change how we approach our relationship to exercise?

When can we stop doing, and start being? Being present in the moment, being present in our bodies, feeling our bodies move and a connection to our mind and body? When can we stop seeking the doing - stop the need to feel pain after an exercise class? Since when was it such a good thing to be in pain for days after a Pilates class because we worked our abs so much? I had this very conversation with a new client recently. After her first class, she was explaining that this new way of working was strange to her - her whole experience with exercise has been to finish a class dripping with sweat, being pushed by personal trainers to maximum muscle fatigue. Whilst she found many exercises in the class challenging, her mindset has yet to make the shift away from no pain, no gain.

Lederman states in his paper, *The Myth of Core Stability*, that "Continuous and abnormal patterns of use of the trunk muscles could be a source of potential damage for spinal or pelvic pain conditions." If you were to run for a bus and wake up the following day in so much pain you couldn't walk, I think you might be concerned. I know I would! So why is it acceptable and positively encouraged in many Pilates classes? Was it really what Joseph Pilates was calling for with his method of Contrology? He actually states in his book *Return to Life* "There really is no need for tired muscles." He recommends 3 repetitions of some of his exercises in the *Classical Mat* - with only a couple rising to a maximum of 12 repetitions with practice. What would he make of this over-recruitment, over-repetition environment so that clients feel the burn? Pilates wanted us to "build a sturdy body and sound mind fit to perform every daily task with ease and perfection." I have read and reread his book and I cannot find any reference from him to 'feel the burn.' He wanted no pain, no strain! He wanted natural movement.

I believe it is because we feel we need to be doing - if we do curl-ups or roll-ups in a class, we should really *do* them, or else we're not working hard enough, right? If it doesn't hurt I clearly have not been working hard enough! Why? My two young children run around the park, jumping, climbing trees, playing football - they don't have any expectations of experiencing pain. They must move, effortlessly. If they were in pain the following day, again, I would be concerned. I would be at the doctor's surgery with them!

My Integral Movement Method foundation is to remove this no pain, no gain attitude and replace it with no pain, no strain. Why do we want to add strain and tension to our bodies when we can achieve the same, if not more, without it? Life can be stressful enough - why do we want to add more stress at the very time when we could be nurturing and strengthening ourselves to deal with these very stresses? We end up in an endless stress cycle. When I start working with clients on my Integral Movement Method, we begin by unwinding, undoing what was in place before. This will be explained in Chapter Seven in greater detail. I refer to it as reprogramming the body. When we have been submerged in this doing mentality for a long time, often many adult years, this has become our habit, who we are. Our nervous system has been on high alert - in the fight or flight mode. Fight or flight is our primal response to danger - it would save your life if you were being chased by a bear. Adrenalin is pumped through the body, giving you the power to run really fast if you had to. However, as a long-term strategy in your daily life today, it does not serve you well. It is not necessary for healthy functioning of the body. If the adrenal glands work in overtime, we can never switch off, always feeling like we are about to run for our lives. In his book, *Return to Life*, Joseph Pilates was clearly expressing the same thoughts, stating "this too fast pace is plainly reflected in our manner of standing, walking, sitting, eating ...... our nerves being on edge from morning to night." That was in 1945 - I wonder what he would think today in the age of online streaming, smartphones, access to anything 24/7!

If you take this attitude or mindset to your Pilates class, you are going to be seeking this high response, the pain of doing something, to feel the burn. My Integral Movement Method is often met with questioning, resistance and reluctance from people who are used to working in a doing mentality. Given time, what we see is an ability to harness a different way of moving through trying less, squeezing less, releasing more. I attended a class with Pilates guru Alan Herdman in London and he stated "The harder an exercise becomes the easier it should look." I repeat this phrase often to my clients - it really helps portray the point that how will an exercise ever look easy, effortless and fluid if you have a laboured breathing pattern, are visibly straining in your face and body to achieve the move. There is a different way, a new unexplored movement strategy within you that your body is craving to use.

All I ask is to give your body time; listen to your body. The wonderful news is that these patterns of moving are already within your body - it does not have to be mentally learnt like an aerobics routine. All we have to do is uncover it. When clients first come to a session or a class, we have to retrain the body to move out of this state. If a client has been ill or recovering from injury, or is a chronic pain sufferer, movements will already be guarded, protected and nerves will be over-sensitised. So this work is essential and potentially life-changing.

Through the Integral Movement Method we are returning to the natural movement patterns we had as children, where we move effortlessly, freely. As we have already looked at in Chapter Three, everything is connected. So this fluid movement cannot be just a physical response. It is everything. When it is everything, there is no internal conflict; your body is happy to move. It is beautifully responsive rather than fighting you back. It is not about doing a spine curl to do an exercise. If you allow it, if you invest the time to mentally train and re-programme your brain for it, you will start to move in a totally new way.

We aim to leave behind the no pain, no gain attitude. We move onto a strain free existence where we learn to Do Less, Gain More.

CHAPTER SIX
DO LESS, GAIN MORE

In this chapter, we really start to see the full picture - we are aiming to remove the stresses and tension from the body to unveil a freer, lighter version of you. A person with complete body awareness, the ability to participate in daily activities with ease whilst feeling strong and in control, mentally and physically.

So how do we do less but gain more? Vanda Scaravelli stated "It is not so much the performance of the exercises that matters but how we approach them mentally and physically." I am in such agreement with this. I work with clients of all ages - the youngest being 10 through to the oldest over 90. That is a huge range. The 10 year old is most likely going to be doing different exercises to the 90 year old (although I never assume anything and have seen amazing things). The point is - do I really mind if the 90 year old cannot perform the exercise to the same ability than the 10 year old? Absolutely not. It is not about what it looks like. Obviously there are certain things that go without question, like client safety and alignment, but I have and always will be looking at the integrated movement quality. It is quality over quantity in my classes and sessions. I would rather have 3 repetitions performed well than 20 repetitions rushed through for the sake of doing the exercise.

Integrated movement quality to me is putting all the elements of these chapters together. I am looking for a response from within before and during a movement from the body I am working with. Robert Schliep (Fascia in Sport and Movement) talks of "the ease and flow of the breath and the subtle ability to transmit the breathing motion through the whole pose and body rhythmically." Further he states "There is no need for extraneous, unnecessary tightness, floppiness or strain." This is how we can move when we tune in, when we work with our fascia, our whole integrated body.

We have talked in detail about how the breath is integral to everything; we have spent time feeling and questioning our body's responses to gravity. We are by now really beginning to view our body differently as a whole unit. Do we have the mental and physical connections working together? At the beginning of a session, I often ask clients to show me their execution of a simple exercise. At this stage, I am simply looking for what movement patterns are in place. How do they move? Remember the key takeaway number 2, there is no right or wrong. Whatever you have been doing, your body has adapted beautifully to allow you to move every day. But, can we improve that process, especially if that process is now presenting you with pain, discomfort and restrictions? I had a client come to see me who was experiencing terrible hip pain, to the point that hip replacements were being discussed with the surgeons. Upon observing his static and moving posture, it was apparent that he did not put any weight on the left side of his body. When he stood and walked, he was positively avoiding the left side (which is where he had more hip pain). The body had adjusted his patterns to walk and function every day - but was now subconsciously avoiding any weight bearing on the left side. He was totally unaware of this fact and we started to work together to bring initial awareness back to this side of his body. That alone is a huge step - the brain starts to recognise that a whole new world of movement does still exist. Over time, if the body does not feel threatened by this reintroduction, balance to the body can be recovered.

When we become aware of what we are doing, we can make a change. If we are not aware of what movements we do that could be compromising our system - like my client above - we probably will not change it. Not because we do not want to - nobody wants to be in pain or discomfort or be inhibited from playing a sport because of a shoulder injury, for example. Without awareness, your brain will assume this current way is fine and will continue repeating the pattern over and over. If this is a faulty movement pattern, one that either gives pain already or one that over time will lead to the onset of pain, the body will continue to do it because the brain knows no difference. Your brain is the control centre and has all the final decisions on movement - whether they are safe or threatening to do. If we can communicate with the brain in a way it perceives as non-threatening, we can begin the reprogramming.

For example, if every time I stood up out of a chair I arched my back and used my lower back to pull me up, my lower back muscles could start to get irritated and annoyed by this. They would feel unsupported in their 'tent' set up (see Chapter Two). If I continued to do this for 20 years, I could have a pretty rigid set pattern in my body that I would not even be aware of, until a movement therapist points it out and I change the pattern by relearning and reprogramming to remove the element of that action that could be causing the discomfort in my back.

I gave the example above of standing up from a chair because it is what we do many times every day. It is an issue for many people - getting up out of a chair without back pain. You will notice on the Integral Movement Method exercises that many are standing ones as you progress. There reason for this is: a) It is functional - it is where we spend most of our day - upright. We need to be able to be here, so let's learn to be here without pain or discomfort. That's going to be life-changing in itself. Imagine being able to go for a walk or attend a drinks party and stand without a nagging backache. b) Many people have lost the ability to use their legs effectively. As we have discussed in earlier chapters, this is largely due to our lifestyle today. We sit down an awful amount of time. Our arms probably do more work than our legs. Take a moment to think about your average day. What percentage of time do you use your legs - walking, running, climbing stairs, jumping, squatting? What percentage of time do you use your arms - chopping, cutting, computer, smartphone, reading, carrying, and swinging from trees? Yes, swinging from trees! Our ancestors, of course, would have spent time doing activities such as climbing and hanging around from trees - as well as running, jumping and squatting. They didn't have comfortable sofas to slouch back on in the evening after a day tapping away on their computer. They would have been in much better shape than us physically. They used their legs and their arms in a balanced way. A typical person today does not. But that's why I love my job because I get to reintroduce people to their legs. We do this with a variety of exercises, as you will discover in the foundation programme in Chapter Nine, but guess what - we always start with the feet! Remember how important the feet are in everything that goes on further up your body. So, through those exercises you have already covered, and many more, we wake up the feet. The more secure your feet feel, the more secure the rest of your body will feel. You will have to do less work further up - that's your tight lower back muscles or shoulder muscles you are using to hold yourself up every day! Work on that image of the tree from Chapter Two - you will be amazed at how much freer you start to feel. You start to use your legs as they were designed. - a supportive structure from which the rest of the body can rest lightly.

When I first trained with Polestar Pilates in London in 2010, I had the very same issue. Remember, I had come from a place of zero body awareness, hanging off my joints, holding tension constantly, and letting go was a whole new experience to me. I had come a very long way when I started my comprehensive studio apparatus training, but there is always more to learn. The training at Polestar Pilates is intense and extremely challenging, mentally and physically. Whenever I performed an exercise, I was told to get into my legs. Whether I was upright on a reformer, practising Swan over the barrel, anything - legs, legs, legs was called out to me. To hear this cue sparked something in my brain - it was as though the mere fact I had legs I could use was a new phenomenon to my brain. Second, my sensory nervous system went into action to try and figure out what exactly was meant by this. It was new! My brain loved that. Gradually, I started to get it. The more I did with my legs, the less I had to do with my spine, my shoulders, my arms, my neck - whatever it was I had previously been doing all the work with! Those areas were now not being overused and started to free up. I felt better; less aches, less headaches. I felt different - I distinctly remember one occasion learning a standing exercise on the Reformer called Scooter. I had to be tactically guided into how to move my legs in my hip socket. I exclaimed "I've never moved like that ever." So I started to find a balance. It was revolutionary to me - I had got into such a habit of using my front body and arm and shoulder domination, I had lost my integrated body. My pre-Pilates life had been a sedentary one of life in the City of London - sitting down 90% of my day using a computer. To have the opportunity to share this knowledge and experience with my clients - and now you - is fantastic.

For most people it is not an overnight fix - some people do pick concepts and feelings up immediately, but for most of us there is a certain degree of unwinding to do, relearning, experiencing new sensations. That in itself can be scary too - to feel new sensations. Maybe you have come from a place of pain where the thought of movement is fearful. Or maybe you are coming from a place of high achievement where you are used to pushing and achieving at all costs. There is nothing wrong with achievement - brilliant. I am all for it - I consider myself a high achiever too, but can we also balance that out with a little mindful, quiet, reflective time? I work long hours, I have a young family and busy Pilates studio to manage, but I can go to this 'other place' to find my balance, my focus, my clarity. You maybe have had little time or room or inclination until now to let in new space into your life. But to move on, we need to make room - time, patience, experiencing, being.

You may be thinking this sounds like a very slow process. And initially it is - absolutely, deliberately so. With the Integral Movement Method, it is all about the thoughtful movement. Warning for the high achievers reading this - you are going to dig deep into your patience and persistence qualities. But I am guessing that's what made you a high achiever in the first place! Let's utilise it. When we move slowly, we watch, we listen, we observe. We take time to notice what we are doing, what we are feeling. The brain registers this as something new - remember my experience with discovering my legs. When performed slowly, the brain registers this as something unthreatening, so it is more likely to accept a change. Have you ever driven from your house to the supermarket and cannot remember driving there? You have no recollection of changing gear, turning roundabouts. That's because your brain was on automatic pilot. It tuned out. It did not recognise this as something new and did not pay attention. We do not want this while we are reprogramming and relearning how to move with less strain so that we can move better and feel great. Scaravelli says "To be sensitive is to be alive." We cannot access sensitivity if we are operating on automatic pilot. I am not saying that the exercises will always be performed at a slow pace. I have no objection to exercises being performed at a challenging pace ONCE these foundations have been established. The Pilates mat and reformer classes I teach regularly at the studio to my advanced students and competitive sports people are challenging, advanced work. I work with elite sports people as well as rehabilitation clients. This method works from one end of the spectrum to the other. I have had the pleasure of working with a client who is a marathon runner and triathlete and a high achiever. He was encouraged to come to Pilates by his wife as he was experiencing regular injuries with his tough training schedule. Over the course of a year we worked on his approach, less push, slowing down. We noticed a marked change not only in his flexibility, agility and elasticity, but also his injuries diminished. He completed his first marathon in just 3 hours 2 minutes without injury. As for his triathlon performance, his fellow athletes have commented on his improved times - asking him what bike has he bought, what new gear has he got that has created this change. My client says "I've been doing Pilates." The response was "No really, what new bike have you got?" There was a certain amount of disbelief that the change had come about not from a new bike, but from attending a weekly Pilates class which had taken out the elements of no pain, no gain and replaced it with do less, gain more. This client is now training for an IronMan!

The Integral Movement Method is subtle work. Through the initial slowness, the body will accept this new way of working, so that the advanced Pilates repertoire is performed with grace and fluidity. Remember Alan Herdman's quote from the previous chapter about harder exercises looking easier. Having said that, the ability for a client to perform an exercise such as a ribcage closure or knee fold with total awareness, with no visible force or effort, is the sign of an advanced practitioner, in my eyes. I have seen the advanced classical mat performed in a manner of squeeze and push and pull, with limbs almost disconnected from the body. So much effort exerted to get the job done, ego proud to master the Classical Mat.

Joseph Pilates in his book, *Return to Life,* speaks of moving with "minimum effort." He describes his exercises as "correctly executed and mastered to the point of subconscious reaction." This ability to move with ease, without tension in a subconscious manner, is our ultimate aim. It is what he had prescribed. I fear it has been lost somewhere through the years with the boot-camp style so-called Pilates classes that have emerged to feed this demand of "doing."

Take a test. You will only ever find true release and length when "the pushing and pulling have come to an end." (Scaravelli, Awakening the Spine) Scaravelli felt that if we are not relaxed when we are working, we are not lengthening. The job of your spine is to find space and elongation. It does not seek compression and shortening.

EXERCISE - LENGTHEN YOUR HAMSTRINGS

This is a traditional exercise you will often see performed by people at the end of an exercise class. I was also taught this particular hamstring exercise as part of my initial Pilates mat based training in 2007 – the aim being to stretch the hamstrings whilst anchoring the back down. People always think they have short hamstrings (or maybe they are too long - muscles can feel tight and sore if they are too short or too long). You will need a stretch band for this exercise.

Lie on your back and place the band around one foot (see Fig 9). Hold the band with both hands at the end. Simply straighten the leg and attempt to lengthen the leg. Notice how straight the leg goes, how it feels in your hamstrings and pelvis, lumbar spine.

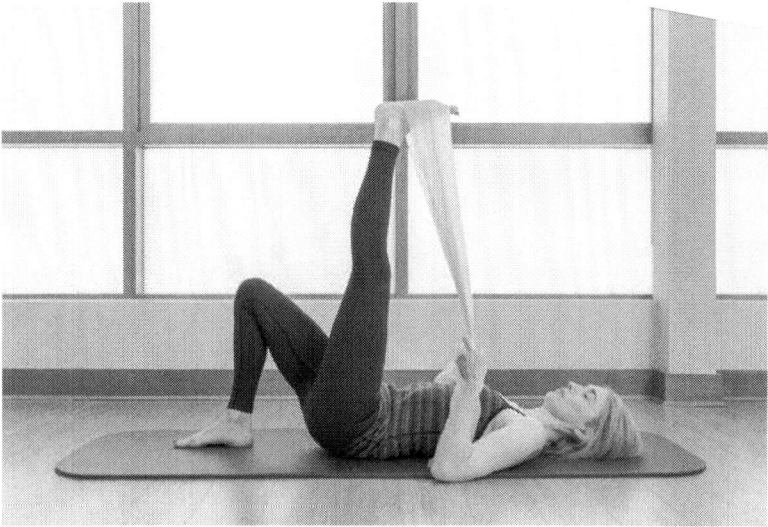

Fig 9

Lower the leg down by bending the knee first. Switch to the other leg and see how that side feels. Make a mental note of how each leg felt.

In her book, Scaravelli speaks of a similar exercise performed without a band 'Reclining Big Toe Pose'. With her version, the movement is initiated with the breath, using the exhale to gain length in the spine which allows the leg to be free. I particularly like how she speaks of moving in "little round movements" so as not to force the leg to lengthen. I call it 'teasing' the body to lengthen. Can we achieve a more effective result with an approach like Scaravelli's?

Return the band to the first foot and we will approach the exercise again.

This time start with the knee bent (see Fig 10). Feel the weight of your thigh bone resting in the hip socket. Soften the hip, feel the weight of the pelvis under you. Slowly start to uncurl the leg, but only allowing the leg to uncurl as a response to the weight of the thigh bone. Every time you exhale, allow the thigh bone to sink a little deeper into the hip socket. Feel every time it sinks, the hip socket becomes a little wider. There is more room for the thigh bone to slide inside. Allow the thigh bone to rotate from left to right as you continue to uncurl the leg with every out-breath. The out-breath will be quiet, slow and measured.

Slowly and gradually, notice the spiralling as the leg gets longer - the calf gets lighter as the thigh gets heavier. The back of the knee unfolds creating space here too behind the knee joint. Continue this until the leg has unravelled (see Fig 11). It does not matter if you cannot fully straighten the leg - that is not the objective of the exercise. Make a mental note of how that exercise felt compared to the first one and then repeat on the other leg.

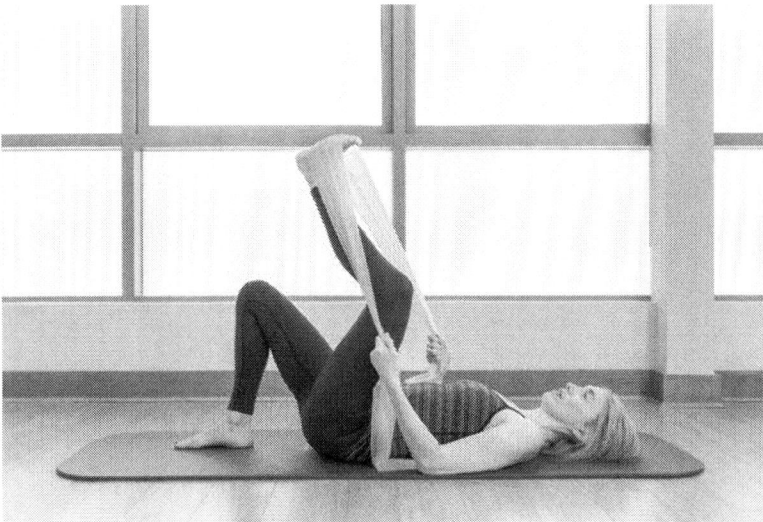

Fig 10

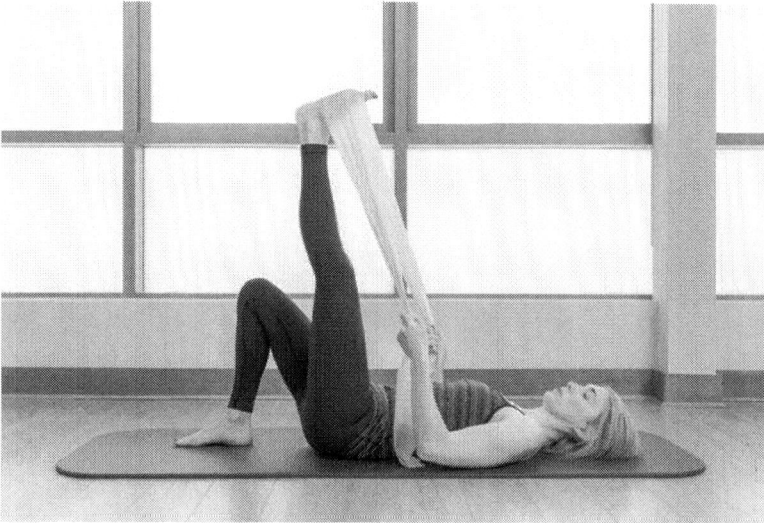

Fig 11

Can you observe from the photographs (Fig 9) that version 1 of the hamstring stretch has a hyperextended knee with a sense of rigidity around the pelvis? Compare this to the softer image of version 2 (Fig 11) - the knee is soft, the pelvis is weighted down and yet the leg still has the ability to extend. The missing element is the tension. Tension has been removed from version 2, allowing greater freedom in the joint space.

POST EXERCISE QUESTIONS

- Which one felt more comfortable?
- Did you go further the second time?
- Did you notice less resistance the second time?
- How did the breath play a part in the exercises?
- Did the breath help facilitate a greater movement potential?
- How do you think you could apply this approach to other exercises or stretches you currently do?

Through the second version of the same exercise, we were not just engaging the hamstrings - the title of the exercise could have misled you. But maybe you realised that because you now know from previous chapters that everything is connected and we cannot isolate individual muscles. If you do like stretching as part of your exercise routine, it is worth approaching it in this less aggressive way to the tissue. Robert Schliep in his book *Fascia in Sport and Movement* reminds us that "If we force a stretch, then the ability of the tissues to restore might be compromised."

What does he mean by compromised? Apart from soft tissue damage like overstretching, maybe causing a tear or strain, I believe he is referring to the concept of elasticity. It is not just about how much we can stretch or be flexible, but rather the ability for the tissue to bounce back from that stretch. He seeks a "suitable balance between stiffness (resistance to deformation) and elasticity (the ability to reform the original shape)." I explain this rather technical aspect to my clients using one of the springs from the Pilates apparatus. For example, I can pull on the spring and increase the tension in the spring. But when I let go, there is enough 'good tension' in the spring for it to bounce back to its original length. It looks exactly the same as it did before. It is good for the spring to be pulled and expanded on a regular basis because if I didn't, the spring could get over-stiff, rusty, possibly break when I tried to use it. It would not be a healthy spring. The other extreme, however, is if I kept pulling the spring so that the coils start to unravel, and when let go, the coils had then changed shape permanently and could never bounce back. I have changed its function, its ability to move well permanently, its agility, its strength. We do not want to be the spring that cannot bounce back! We do not want to be the spring that becomes rusty and stiff through underuse and inactivity. We want to move with ease and grace, expanding and contracting when we want to suit whatever force we are putting through the body at that time. We want to be light, bouncy and responsive.

At the studio, I work with sports people - tennis players, golfers, runners and skiers predominantly. We work hard together to give them the flexibility they need to rotate, extend, flex but we also work on the ability for them to find their elastic recoil. We do not work on just flexibility. If we did, they would end up like the spring that cannot bounce back. We work on building their tent (Chapter Three). An organisation that has enough 'good tension' inside that creates space within the body to move freely; an organisation that can rotate quickly and fluidly when hitting a tennis ball for example; an organisation that has enough recoil to bounce back from hitting the tennis ball easily and with the minimum amount of effort back to its original form, ready to hit the next ball. When it looks easy, we are really connected. I always refer to players like Roger Federer - how easy can a man make tennis look? He is a perfect example of balance between strength and elasticity giving us agility, grace and ease of movement.

I use this same methodology with all my clients, though, and this is what I am also sharing with you now. It works for everyone, not just elite sports people. In whatever degree you need it in your daily life, you can achieve the appropriate amount of elasticity. It will not be the same requirement as an elite tennis player - most of us do not need that - but we want to be able to function well every day and play the sports or activities we want to without pain or restriction. That's what this Integral Movement Method will give you.

KEY MESSAGE NO 7 - THE LESS I PUSH AND FORCE, THE MORE FREEDOM AND SPACE I CREATE

KEY TAKEWAY NO 8 - WHEN I FORCE, MY MUSCLES SHORTEN - I CREATE THE OPPOSITE RESULT OF WHAT I WANTED IN THE FIRST PLACE

With all the background now in place, we are in a position to move onto the Integral Movement Method in detail. Are you ready to change your movement patterns forever? We begin with the mental preparation.

CHAPTER SEVEN
THE INTEGRAL MOVEMENT METHOD:
THE MENTAL PREPARATION

As you have probably realised by now, this is not a boot-camp style exercise routine. It is an intelligent form of movement - one where you will be listening and working with your body in harmony, minus the stresses and strains. The problem many of us have in our daily lives is that sheer amount of information, and demands upon us. Our minds are full of chit-chat. Our minds are well-trained to distract us with thoughts, feelings, fears, what ifs, to do lists all the time - if we allow it. That is the key. You do not have to allow it - you can be in complete control of your thoughts and direct them as you wish. You have a choice. Have you ever experienced a really bad day? You know the ones where you wake up and it's raining, there's no hot water for a shower, no milk in the fridge, your train is late, you get splashed by a passing car with a puddle and so on. You can end up spiralling into thoughts of why me, this is a terrible day, I hate days like this and things generally keep going in that direction. You cannot wait for the day to be over! But, I bet you've also experienced truly fantastic days. Days where you wake up and it's raining, there's no hot water for a shower, no milk in the fridge, your train is late, and you get splashed by a passing car and so on! And yet you just let it wash over you. It didn't bring you down. The exact same day - one day you hate it, you resent it, and another day you feel so positive, so engaged, so motivated, so calm and undistracted by all the irritations life can throw at you that it just does not matter. You are in the zone. You are in a different state mentally. Wouldn't it be great if you could harness this power every day? Imagine days where your internal chit-chat - I call them my little voices that tell me I cannot do this and I haven't got time - has slowed right down. You can turn them off when you want to. You can tune out and zone in. The physical effect this has on your body will be amazing too. Remember we said back in Chapter Three that the fascia was the largest organ for proprioception in the body? Well, your fascia is affected by every single thought and feeling you have. If you feel down, miserable, negative much of the time, the fascia is going to respond accordingly. Tightening up, responding to you. How do you think it would respond if you felt great, positive much of the time? You could probably 'jump for joy.' Maybe that's where that expression came from!

So, let's do it. Let's train our minds to quieten down so that we can tune into our bodies quicker and easier when we come to do the exercises and when we approach real-life situations and events. The Integral Movement Method requires reassessing and reflecting. You will not be in the right frame of mind to do that if your mind is whizzing all over the place. Here are some examples that you can do at any quiet time of your day. These are some of my favourites that I use with clients. There are three versions - lying, sitting and standing, so whether you are in a crowned tube train or in the dentist chair, you will be able to still the mind. The more you practise and play with these visualisations, the stronger the mind will become. You will be able to bring yourself back from getting into the sometimes potentially damaging internal dialogues we have with ourselves and bring about a more positive frame of mind. State of mind is everything to what you can and will achieve. As the example above of the type of day you can have - the days were the same, but the state of mind was different. Despite the setbacks and irritations, the second example still came out feeling undeterred. The first one was dragged down. Which one do you want to be?

1) Lying Down on Your Back - Supine

Assume a relaxation position with knees bent or legs long. Allow the eyes to close and the eyeballs to soften and fall gently back inside the head. Take notice of your body resting on the mat - how much contact you are making right now and observe, as though you were standing over your own body watching. Turn your attention to your left foot, your left little toe and allow the bones to soften, the joints to open. Continue this through all the toes - first drawing your attention to that toe, really visualise the toe in your mind and feel it soften. Work your way through the toes and then start to work up the foot - saying each part of the body to yourself in your mind. You do not need to be anatomically technical - whatever works for you. So, you will have the sole of the foot, the ankle, the shin, the calf, the knee, the thigh. You then start again on the right foot and so on. Each body part will become softer, heavier, released as you work through your body.

If you have a particular area where you have been experiencing discomfort or pain, spend more time there. Let the mind rest there; see if you can quieten that area down with your breath, creation of space, and release. Continue through the pelvis, the spine, the internal organs, ribs, collarbone, sternum, arms (including all the fingers), neck, jaw, ears, forehead, and hair.

Once you have worked your way up your body from your feet to your hair, notice how you feel. Does it feel an effort to even think about moving even your little finger? Are you aware of every single part of your body? Does it feel alive? Is there any tingling in the body as blood starts to flow?

Spend a few moments, or as long as you have, enjoying this moment of peace and release and a quiet mind. The mind will have slowed down. This is a beautiful exercise to do if you are struggling to sleep too.

2) Seated in a Chair - Feet Flat on the Floor

It is very important for this exercise that your feet are flat on the floor and you are seated in a peak state - that means no slumping or slouching. You are ready to receive. Hands can rest in your lap.

Allow the eyes to close. Gently rock forward and backward on your pelvis to check you are in fact sitting on your sit bones, not back on your sacrum or tailbone. We are looking for the place that feels heavy and comfortable in the pelvis. Notice the feet in contact with the floor, feel the weight of your feet. Do not hold onto your legs, rather let them rest into the ground. Allow the thigh bones to rest on the chair so that the skin of the legs is soft and drapey. The thigh bone drops to the back of the leg, resting heavy, no longer held in place. The legs feel heavy, the pelvis rests on the chair. From the waist down you feel weighted. Notice the spine's response to this weightiness. It almost starts to hover above the pelvis with free-flowing breath. The abdominals are no longer squashed by a slouched position. Continue to feel the weight of the legs with each exhale, and the opposition of lightness from the spine. Allow the arms to rest on the spine, like you were wearing a very heavy velvet cloak. The cloak drapes over your shoulders, down your arms and the material gathers at the back of your pelvis.

From this peak state, begin to draw with every out-breath a bright light down through the body, filling every cell with light and space. Depending on how you are feeling when you do this exercise, the white light can represent anything. If you are in pain or sick, this can be a healing light.   If you are tired after a long day, an energising light. If you are stressed and nervous, a calming light. Whatever you need. Draw the light down to your feet and into the ground. Then draw it back from the ground, up the legs and out of the top of the head.

The body feels enveloped in this bright white light. Every cell is vibrating with this white light. Notice how you feel. Tingling? Warmth? Space? Notice whatever comes to you. Notice the mind - did it stop its chit chat for a few minutes? As you open your eyes, do you feel refreshed or calm? If you did this at your desk for a few moments, do you feel a greater clarity and focus to continue your work? Try to continue this seated posture at your work station.

3) Standing in a Balanced Way

Assume a standing posture as we learnt together in Chapter Two. Begin the visualisation at your feet, assess the connection and spread of the feet into the ground. Assess balance side to side and front and back. As you find your centre, allow the breath to respond and change to this. Allow the breath to come to you rather than sucking in the air. Be breathed. Notice the subtle pauses between each breath before the body draws it back in. This will quieten the mind remarkably as you simply observe this natural response.

From here, visualise you are standing on a fountain of bubbling water. Feel the bubbles tickling your feet, the energy of the water. Allow the water to travel upwards through the body - through the entire body, flowing upwards with direction and energy. You feel the body filling with water, supporting you from the inside out. The water continues through the spine, through the neck and out of the top of your head. Feel the power of the upward force through your centre, lengthening the spine, lifting the pelvis off the top of the thighs so that the pelvis almost floats.   Then, simply allow the water to cascade down the outside of your body, like you were under a gentle shower. Soft caress to the skin, touching every cell, all the way down to the floor.   There are no sharp edges, just a softness to your outline. We are left with a strong centre with a visible softness on the outside.   No taut, tense muscles but a soft, fluid, lean muscle.   The strength comes from within.   This is the beauty - you feel strong on the inside, but without the bulk on the outside. You may look soft and gentle, but a warrior lies within!

These three exercises will soon be available as a bonus in audio - visit my website www.pilateswithouttears.com and register your interest to receive your introduction package on a series of online classes coming soon. Be one of the very first to receive these additional bonuses as soon as they are released to the public.

Continue to practice these as much as you can until they become part of you, the place where you can access the mental strength and physical connection when you need it - not just in your Pilates class, but anytime, anywhere.

Let's now explore the 5-step Integral Movement Method in detail.

CHAPTER EIGHT
THE INTEGRAL MOVEMENT METHOD:
THE 5-STEP STRATEGY

This is it! We have arrived at the detail of The Integral Movement Method - the 5-step no pain, no strain strategy to move and feel great. The great news is it that you will be so prepared for this if you have followed the book through each chapter. This strategy will seem natural to you. Above all, remember, we need to consider all the elements of the process that have come before this for you to be successful and really start to move well and feel great.

The 5 steps are:

- Unwind
- Explore
- Assess
- Refine
- Reflect

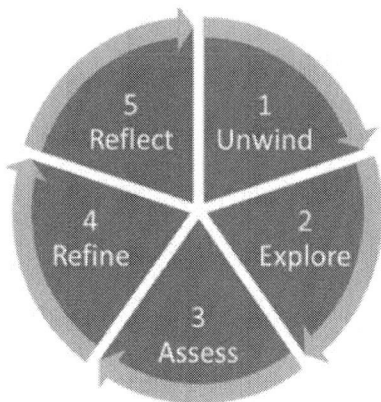

The Integral Movement Method

1. Unwind

This is the first integral step, essential before beginning any exercise. If you are time short, it would still be important for this stage. We need a few moments to close our eyes, observe our breath, switching off our thinking brain. It is your time to start to awaken your sensory awareness. If we jump straight in, we have not shifted mentally from our busy brain to a place where we can really tune in, slow down and observe. If you have rushed from work to a class, then you will still be in 'doing' mode - we are now entering the 'doing less' mode.

Whether you are starting lying or standing, close your eyes. Tune into the rise and fall of your breath. If your mind continues to wander back and forth, keep returning to your breath. You could play with any of the breathing exercises we covered in Chapter One if a guided unwind can assist.

Remember you can download the free audio of those exercises from my website www.pilateswithouttears.com.

Through the process of unwinding, you immediately start to release the tension from the mind and body you may not have been aware you had during the day. Allow your bones, tissues and organs to soften and start creating the space your body craves.

2. Explore

This is where we start to move. I call it explore, because as we discussed it is so much more than doing an exercise. You are exploring your body's potential, your feelings, your power of focus and concentration. At this stage, if you have completed stage one, you will really start to tune in. You will not have time for thinking of your to do list! It is time for movement meditation.

Remember, whether you are new to Pilates or an advanced practitioner, your full participation mentally should be the same. The speed of execution may be different, but the quality should be exactly the same.

We start to move with gravity (as discussed in Chapters One and Two) - moving with the least resistance. We let go to achieve more. In Chapter Nine you will find fifteen exercises with photographs taken from the foundation programme. It will take you through the exercises step by step. As an added bonus, the full programme can be downloaded absolutely free from my website www.pilateswithouttears.com. You will have a complete foundation exercise programme to follow at home with easy, guided instructions.

3. Assess

This is a crucial step - the pause to re-evaluate. We have explored throughout this book the benefits and huge changes we can achieve by observing our body. We have discussed the effect stress and strain can put on the body. This stage is therefore a chance to assess whether you are in fact moving without strain, or you have reverted to an old movement pattern. We pause, we wait, we observe, we shift our mental focus from outside to inside the body.

Typically, you would do 3 or 4 reps of an exercise, observing the body as you do. The key is to look globally, not locally. Sometimes we get so focused on our knee fold or arm opening movement that we are not aware of how the rest of the body is feeling and responding. A typical example would be to clench the jaw muscles in tension or shoulders rising up to the ears causing neck and shoulder discomfort. Or maybe we have stopped breathing altogether. The more you start to observe globally, the more integrated the movements will become. Your body starts to act as a tent - see Chapter Three - as opposed to individual parts moving. Remember, the connective tissue connects everything! The more integrated the movement, the easier it looks and feels.

So a pause - a reassessment is a chance to check in with yourself. If you have been clenching your jaw, it's ok. You just need to recognise that, bring attention to it. Once you have the brain's attention, you can make a change. Most movement issues arise because we are so unaware of what we do. Remember your body does not want to be in pain or stressed. It is designed for survival. Offer it a pain-free, stress-free option and it will take it.

4. Refine

After the pause, we get moving again. We have learnt something neurologically in that reassess - maybe now your jaw muscles will stay soft, your shoulders will drape down your back, your breath will be quiet, deep and full. We continue with the exercises exploring all ranges of movement suitable for us but continuing to observe globally. We may return to the assess stage whenever we feel the need. Again, a full programme of exercises can be downloaded for free as a bonus to you at www.pilateswithouttears.com.

5. Reflect

Always, always include this in your programme. I cannot stress enough the importance to check back in with yourself before you go about your daily activities and busy life. We cannot underestimate the power of this work - you will feel so different to when you started the session. You may feel stronger, calmer, strange - whatever comes to your mind, accept it. What is most important is that you have taken the time to register that something has shifted - mentally, physically. If we do not take this time, we just rush back to our busy schedules on automatic pilot again. We miss a vital opportunity to connect and accept change in awareness into the body.

Complete your last exercise and return to a supine or standing posture. Standing posture is a great way to finish a session during the day as you prepare yourself in an upright, functional position for the day ahead. You will feel amazing, in control, calm and connected - able to face the day's challenges and activities with a renewed focus and energy.

If you are practising towards the end of the day, assume a supine position. The support of the floor will allow you to feel free to relax. Use cushions to support you if needed under the head or pelvis.

Allow yourself to simply notice - notice your breath, your posture, your balance, your weight, whatever you notice. Spend a minimum couple of minutes here up to ten minutes. This should not be a falling asleep moment - you need to stay present and mindful. It is not designed to be a collapse on the floor - it is a relaxed letting go, not a collapse. I like the word surrender as it implies you are giving up all those tensions, restrictions that may have been with you at the start of the session.

You can use the audio from the previous exercises if you prefer a guided exercise. Simply visit the book website www.pilateswithouttears.com to download this free gift.

As you come out of your reflection session, gently allow the eyes to open on your exhale. Encourage a softness to the eyes. Allow the eyes to be soft as you open the eyes - a soft gaze, as opposed to a harsh gaze that we use to look at our computer screens and phones. The softening of the eyeballs alone will release tension around the head and neck. Notice how your peripheral vision has increased as the gaze widens.

Going forward: this is not the end of the journey - this is just the beginning. The more you practice this method, the more you will notice, the more you will become aware of your habits, your posture, your movement.

KEY MESSAGE NO 9 - WHEN I AM AWARE, I CAN MAKE A CHANGE.

Daily activities become easier; exercise and your approach to Pilates begin to change. Energy levels increase as you spend less energy fighting your body by holding tension and making tasks harder than they need to be. Clients find this method simply becomes part of who they are, how they move, how they react to situations. They have learnt to access a calmer state when needed. Let me give you an example. One of my clients was recently at the dentist having a root canal - not a particularly pleasant way to spend a morning. It can be a long process and if you don't like dentists, it can be quite stressful and traumatic. My client was sat in the chair and the dentist began his work. She told me she could hear my voice in her head, guiding her through one of our exercises in the Integral Movement Method. She focused on her breath, she felt the weight of her body and surrendered. Time flew by in the dentist chair and she was able to cope with the whole experience. She remained calm throughout. I was thrilled and honoured to hear that these exercises are seriously helping people in real life.

Most people practice formally in a class 1 to 4 hours a week. That's great - and we are all benefitting from this. But, 4 hours is still short of a full waking week - when you are awake and functioning at work or home. What I envisage and would love everyone to experience is the calm, focused, tension-free, strain-free approach to every hour of your day. And of course you could find you sleep better too when your body is more rested and energy efficient in the day. Clients report experiences where their bodies know how to move in this easy, functional way. I would love everyone to experience this. Life will throw challenges, obstacles and difficulties your way. I am not selling a naïve idea that this method will remove all stress from your life. But what I am offering is a new approach to deal with life's challenges. We have a choice in how we respond and react to what happens to us. You now have a toolbox of techniques, ideas and information that you can use whenever you need them.

Please visit my website www.pilateswithouttears.com to experience some audio and video exercises for free as my gift to you.

CHAPTER NINE
THE INTEGRAL MOVEMENT METHOD EXERCISES

The Foundation Exercises

These exercises are designed to take you in all directions of movement, in a variety of postures from lying down to standing. The later ones are standing, as this is where we spend most of our time - upright. We need to be functional and efficient. I want you to feel comfortable moving in multiple directions because in everyday life that's what you do. We want to be free to twist and turn, spiral and dance with our bodies - rather than moving in guarded or forceful, over-exaggerated ways. These are the foundations, the essence of your movement potential. You are taking the first step. Supportive, easy to master without too much co-ordination or complicated choreography at this stage. This is the first programme - you are going to have time to really focus on these moves - moves that translate to your everyday activities. This is what makes Pilates so fantastic. It is very rarely a pure linear movement - up and down, bending and straightening. A gym routine has mainly linear movements - movements where you push and pull pretty much in one direction. Life is not like that, unless you want to move like a Barbie Doll or Action Man. I hope not! And if you do feel you move like that, now you are really going to explore some fantastic places your body has not been to for a while! Your mind and body have been prepared for this moment. You are so well-tuned that you will be performing these exercises with the minimum amount of muscular effort and yet achieving so much more. Less is More! You will feel when the time is right to move - you will just know. When the breath, the mental and physical body are aligned, you just move. We have gone through an ideal journey through the body together, gaining a deeper understanding of how it works, how it connects, and now we put it into a real exercise programme. This programme deliberately does not have any props or fancy equipment. It does not require a lot of space. I want you to be able to do this at home, or on holiday, or travelling on business.

Below you will see a list of the foundation exercises I have chosen to include in this book. There are of course many exercises to choose from and selection depends very much on the body I am working with. I wanted you to have a rounded selection of exercises here so you can refer back to the steps and background information initially. Refer back whenever you need to, until you really take this into your subconscious.

I also wanted you to have the programme easily accessible on your PC and phone, so I have created a special bonus - a version of all 15 exercises in full colour that you can download and have with you always. This can be downloaded at www.pilateswithouttears.com.

The exercises we will cover here are:

1. Pelvic Roll
2. Supine Arm Rolls
3. Supine Knee Rolls
4. Bridge
5. Supine Rotation
6. Quadruped Hip Softener
7. Prone Baby Extension
8. Side Lying Arm Rolls
9. Side Lying Leg Rolls
10. Standing Side Flexion

11. Standing Forward Roll
12. Standing Hip Softener
13. Ski Feet
14. Standing Knee Roll
15. Standing Arm Roll

Every exercise will guide you through step by step, with photographs. These exercises are very safe and gentle, but as with all exercise programmes, please consult your doctor or medical professional before starting. Please eliminate any exercise that your doctor has told you is not suitable for you for medical or health reasons. Also discontinue any exercise that causes any onset or worsening of pain. Practised regularly, you will start to move differently and feel different. Everyone will respond differently.

Before you begin the programme, please prepare your body by following the exercise examples given in Chapter Seven.

1) Pelvic Roll

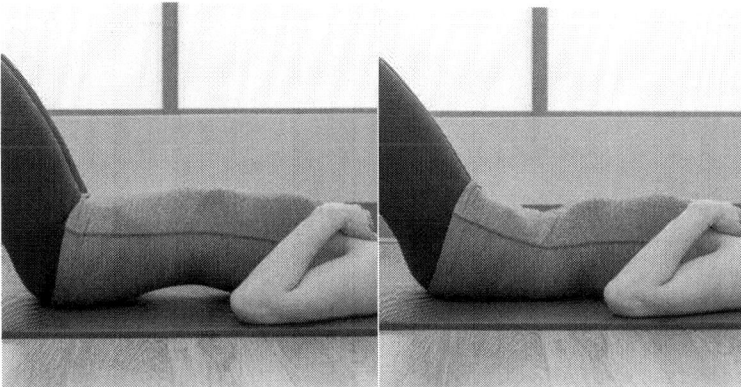

Fig 12

Jeannie Di Bon

Assume your supine position, with knees bent and feet placed flat on the floor in parallel if that does not cause discomfort. Allow the body to settle - recall the earlier exercises where the aim is to allow gravity to soften and give the body a sense of weightiness. Use a head cushion or towel if your neck feels uncomfortable flat on the floor.

Draw your attention to the weight of the back of your pelvis. Can you feel the back of pelvis softening the more time you spend focused on that area? Can you let any holding tension around the hip sockets or buttocks release?

Begin to roll the pelvis forward so that you feel a gentle lifting and arch in your lower back.
Notice how that feels. Allow the pelvis to roll gently backwards until the arch in the back is removed and your lower back is flattened into the floor.

Continue to roll the pelvis forward and backwards. You can place your hands on your hip bones if that helps give you a sense of movement in that area.

As you get familiar with the rolling action, start to introduce the breath so that the breath facilitates the move itself. As you inhale, can you allow the pelvis to be rolled forward by the inflation of the body? The in-breath makes the curves bigger. As you exhale, the breath leaving the body flattens the spine into the floor.

Can you use less muscular effort every time so that the bones are rolling with the breath pattern? Can you get a sense that the pelvis is round so it requires little effort to move? It is perfectly designed for rolling. Allow the body to roll. Allow the pelvis to roll on and off of the thigh bones, without the need for pushing into the floor with your feet or pushing into your lumbar spine.

Allow your pelvis to find a resting place - not too far forward and not too far backward, but somewhere in-between those two range of movements we just explored.   Can you rest with a tension free hip sockets, buttocks and abdomen?

MindBody Connection Moment: How easily can you allow the pelvis to move independently? Are you tempted to push into the pelvis to move it or can you find another way requiring breath and body awareness?

2) **Supine Arm Rolls**

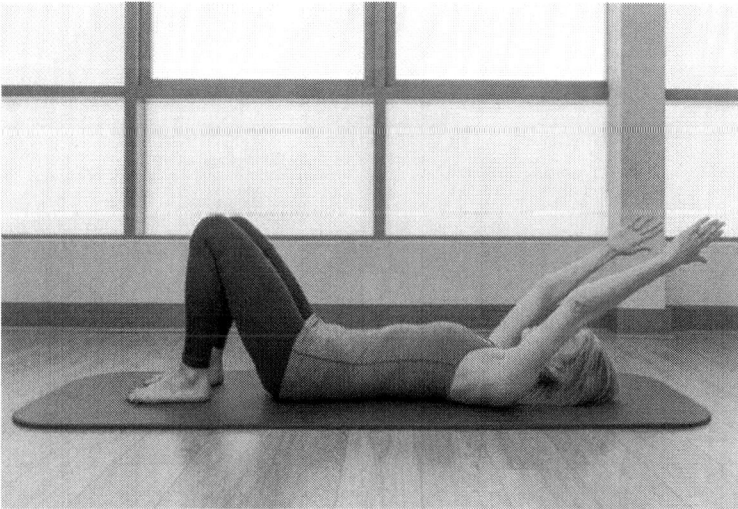

Fig 13

Assume a supine resting position with your arms resting on the floor by your sides.

Find a weighty position of the feet, pelvis, ribs and head. Can you become aware of the back of your body touching the mat? Feel the weight of your shoulders resting on the mat. As you exhale, allow the shoulders to become heavier still. Can the upper arm bones become heavier that the forearm and hand? Can you draw attention to the back of the shoulders dropping down into the floor? As the upper arm bones continue to drop further down, allow the lower arm to float up off the floor until they start to rise above the head and pass over the head towards the wall behind you.

Be more focused on what is going on in the back of the body rather than what the arms are doing. The back of the body includes the soles of your feet. If the arms drift in and out at this stage, do not worry. Be mindful as to what the back of your ribcage, back of pelvis and feet are doing at this moment. Are they still weighted and resting? Take a breath and notice if you can maintain the heaviness into the mat.

On an exhale, allow the arms to slowly float back down to the mat. Do not let them fall but control them with the weight of your body.

Repeat the exercise up to 8 times. Move only from the weightiness of the upper arm bones, so that the upper arm bone is able to roll in the shoulder socket. The top of the arm bone is round and it fits perfectly into the shoulder socket allowing for ease of movement. Can you move without tension in the arms? Be aware of the arms moving from the back of your body so that there is little activity in the front of the shoulders. Allow the torso to rest completely through the whole process. We are trying not to pull the arms up off the floor, but rather roll them backwards in their socket. Pause at any time and let the body sink deeper with an extra out-breath.

MindBody Connection Moment: By maintaining a sense of awareness and weightiness to the back of the body, are you able to move the arms with less effort? Do the arms become lighter as the body becomes heavier?

3) Supine Hip Roll

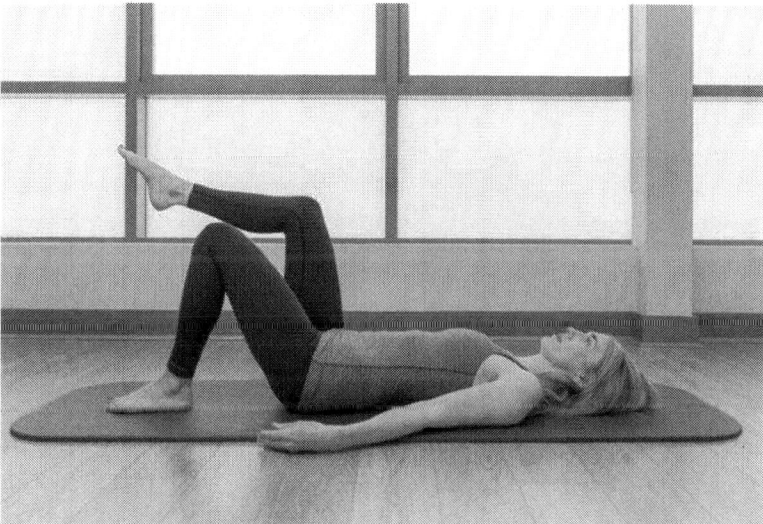

Fig 14

Assume a supine position and establish a sense of heaviness into the floor.

Draw attention to the weightiness of the pelvis. The movement here will be facilitated by the out-breath so take a full deep inhale as discussed in Chapter One. As you exhale, feel the pelvis getting weightier. On the following exhale when you feel the pelvis is at its heaviest, get a sense of one of your legs becoming lighter. So as the torso becomes heavier, can you allow one leg to become lighter? As we sink down into the mat, we can allow the thigh bone to roll into the socket. Again the top of the thigh bone is round and it rolls into the hip socket freely if allowed. Similar to the Arm Rolls, we do not need to lift the leg up off the floor, but rather allow a rolling action in towards the body. The bones are round, the pelvis is round - they are designed to roll together. Look for a sensation of heaviness around the top of the thigh bone so that the knee can feel lighter. Can the tissue of your thigh remain soft and tension-free?

Ideally, the aim is to keep all the body weight into the back of the body, allowing the body to settle so that it can find a lightness to the limb that is moving. Without a sense of heaviness in the torso, there is a greater chance of the lumbar or thoracic spine arching or tensing when the limbs are moving. The torso wants to remain quiet and lengthened, almost undisturbed by the movement of the surrounding limbs.

Hold the position for one breath and, on an exhale, slowly lower the leg down with control. Try not to allow gravity to drop the leg quickly to the floor. Let the leg settle once it meets the floor.

Repeat on the other side and complete 5 repetitions each side.

MindBody Connection Moment: Can you maintain a true sense of weightiness through the back of the body, allowing the lumbar spine to rest quietly as the leg rolls in? Do you notice any tension creeping into the lumbar spine as you move the leg?

These first three exercises have focused on rolling - rolling within joints, rolling bones together thereby reducing muscular effort. Learning to roll maximises movement potential with ease.

4) Bridge

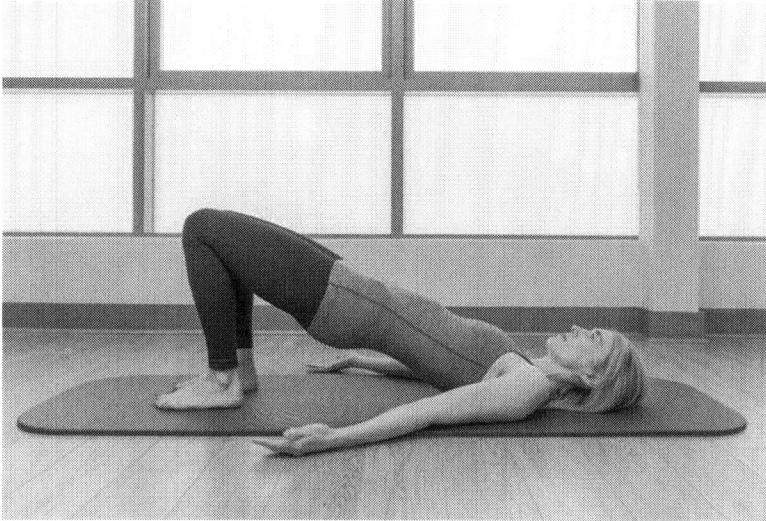

Fig 15

The Bridge requires all those rolling actions come together - it is a global exercise and one that requires a good understanding and appreciation of the role of the feet.

Assume a supine position and settle the body. Ensure your feet are not too far away from the pelvis, with the back of the heels in line with the sitting bones of the pelvis.

As you exhale, feel the weight sinking down through the feet into the floor. It is a sensation of almost making a hole in the floor because of the weight of the feet. As you feel the weight dropping down into your feet, allowing the feet to spread into the floor, can you feel as though the pelvis would like to float off the floor? Is there a sense of the pelvis feeling lighter than the legs and the feet?

The journey into the Bridge comes from the feet, from the weight dropping down into the feet so that the thigh bones are allowed to spiral out of the pelvis and travel away from the weightiness of the head.   The aim is to remove tension from the front and back of the hips - removing any need to squeeze the buttocks. Allow the body to rest between the feet and the shoulders. Allow the front of your body to soften and drop into the back of your body. Touch your abdomen - is it soft?   Can you settle into your feet so that your buttock muscles are not overworking? Allow the front of the hips to open but without being pushed - rather breathe down into the thighs and create space with your breath. Do you feel the spine lengthen when it is not forced to? Create the space with your breath and the body will move into it.

Inhale at the top of the Bridge and begin the journey back down on the exhale. Travel down as you soften the roof of the mouth, the throat, the sternum, the ribcage and pelvis. The pelvis widens as it meets the floor allowing the thigh bone to roll back into the hip socket. Are you able to meet the floor and find your settled position?

Repeat 6 times with the sense of ease increasing each time. Pause and take as many breaths as you need to throughout each Bridge.

MindBody Connection Moment: Where is the balance in the body? Is one part working much more or in isolation to the rest? Can you establish a floating pelvis in between the weightiness of the feet and the shoulders?

5) Supine Rotation

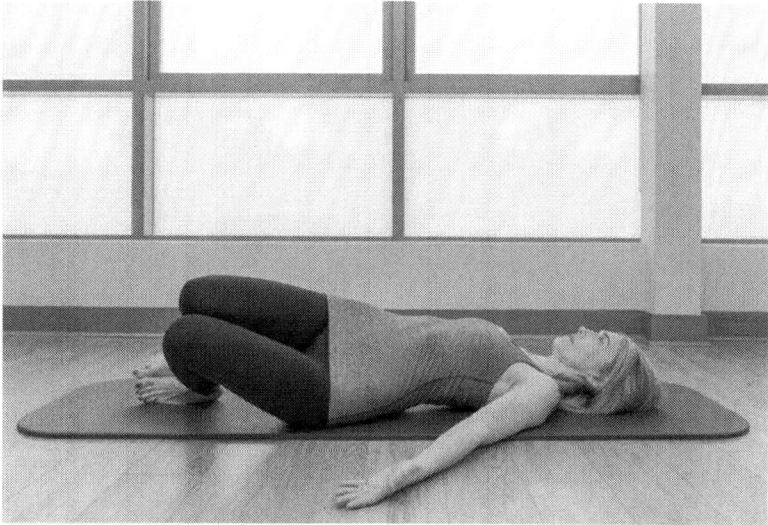

Fig 16

I like to think of the Supine Rotation as a Bridge travelling sideways. It is spinal articulation facilitated by the breath.

Assume a supine position with the feet and knees together and the arms into a small v-shape (wherever is comfortable for your shoulder and neck). Palms face up. Allow the legs to gently connect but try not to squeeze the legs together. Squeezing will simply draw tension in and around the pelvis and inhibit the movement potential. If you were holding a very fine piece of paper between your knees, you would want enough connection not to drop the paper but not enough to rip it.

Use your exhale to roll the pelvis to the side, keeping the opposite shoulder down on the floor. Can you access that sense of weightiness into the head, neck and shoulders so that you are not pushing the shoulder down, but rather it falls backwards to the mat?

Hold the rotation as you inhale. Try to send the breath up into the upper ribcage to expand the tissue and lungs on that side.

As you exhale, feel the weight of the breath drawing the body back to the mat. Try not to pull yourself back to the mat but allow the bones to roll slowly back to the mat. The body is one big spiral - if you allow it, it will unravel itself back to the floor. Can you find your settled position back in the supine position?

Repeat 5 times to each side.

MindBody Connection Moment: Can you move without binding the body down, but encouraging freedom of rolling with the use of the breath? How easily can the body roll from left to right without force?

The prior exercises have all begun on the back where we have the most contact with the floor. This contact with the floor improves our awareness and proprioception of where our body is in space. However, in real life we need to move without continuous tactile feedback and therefore the following exercises start to challenge our awareness and ability to access our sense of weight.

6) Quadruped Hip Softener

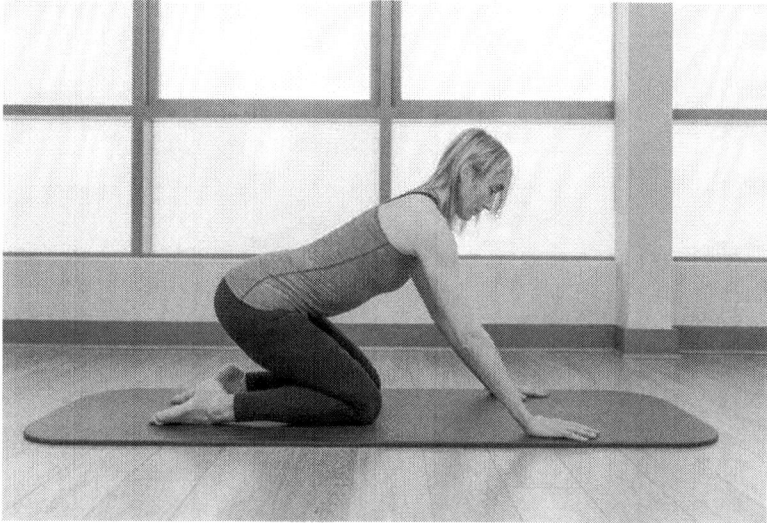

Fig 17

This is our first exercise where we begin in a 4-point kneeling position with pelvis over the knees and shoulders over the hands. We will be moving into the position in Fig 17.

The knees, shins, front of foot and sole of hands are now the only contact points we have with the floor. Our aim is to establish a sense of weightiness into these points. As we have discovered, the more weight that is put into the floor, the lighter and freer the spine becomes. Therefore, allow the weight to fall through the hands and lower limbs, giving the spine a sense of drawing away from the mat. Try to discover your pelvis rolls (Exercise 1) in this position - can you roll your pelvis forward and backwards without disturbing your spine? You can also then establish your resting pelvis in this position - not too far forward so that the spine is rounded and not too far back causing the back to arch.

Once comfortable, allow the front of your hips to soften, almost as though you wanted to create a big crease in the front of your trousers. Allow the body to sink backwards into this crease, but at the same time maintaining the spine long. The spine ideally does not round or arch but maintains a quiet resting place as you move in and out of the hip joints.

As you move backwards, can you get a sense of the breastbone sliding forwards? Can the shoulders and arms rest tension-free? There is no pushing with the arms to move backwards, but rather softening into the hip. Can you breathe easily in this position? If you have any knee pain or prior injury - please keep the range of knee flexion to a position that is comfortable.

When you are ready to return, use an exhale to drop weight further down into the shins and hands and draw the body forward and up at the same time.

Repeat 8 times.

7) Prone Baby Extension

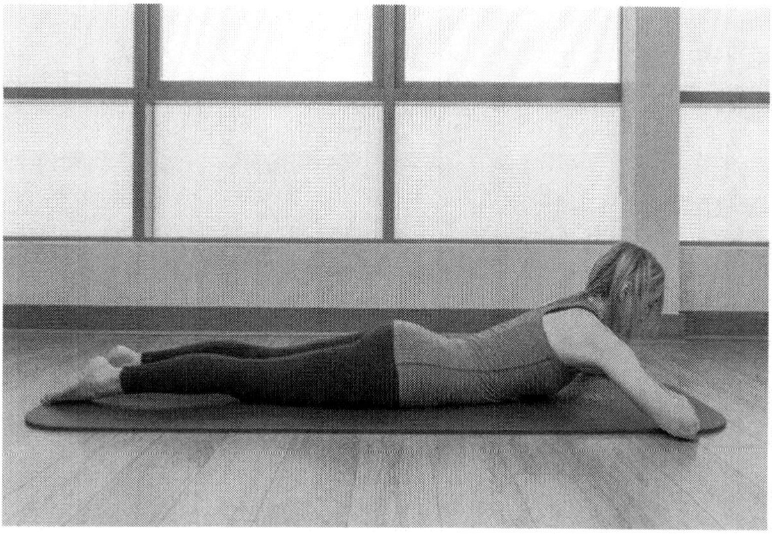

Fig 18

Following the Bridge and the Quadruped, the spine will be better prepared for extension from the floor. As this is our first exercise lying prone, take a few moments to rest your head in your hands and feel the weight of your body sinking into the floor. If your lower back feels uncomfortable, you can place a cushion under the front of the hips to support the back. It is really important that the lower back is pain-free during extension. Please listen to your body. This exercise is not about height - as you can see from the Fig 18, most of the ribcage is still resting on the floor.   It is a small amount of extension.

Once you have established a sense of resting on the front of the body, draw your attention to the breath. Notice how the exhale allows the body to sink deeper into the floor. We are again aiming to allow the parts of the body that stay in contact with the floor to remain heavy, while the moving parts feel lighter. This is created with the breath.

With that in mind, allow the legs to feel weightier with every exhale. From the pelvis down to the feet, can you get a sense of leaving the legs resting on the floor? It is as though the thigh bones themselves are weighted down. With every exhale, can you allow the upper body to begin to float up - ideally without pushing into the arm bones? The arms and shoulders are resting into the floor, allowing the spine the freedom to move between the shoulder blades. There will of course be weight falling into the arm bones, but try to avoid the temptation to push up with your arms. This is not a press up exercise. We are establishing a lightness in the spine to extend forward and up simultaneously.

The number of exhales is not important, neither is the height of your extension. Every body is different. The most important element is your breath and giving your weight to the floor. If you back is not used to extending, please ensure your lower back does not feel pinched. Keep the height low and away from pain free areas until the tissue becomes more elastic.

Once you have reached your extension, take an inhale allowing the lungs to expand. As you exhale, slowly allow the spine to settle back down onto the mat.

Repeat 5 times.

MindBody Connection Moment: Where is the breath and how can you utilise it to allow the spine to lighten and float away from the mat?

8) Side lying arm roll

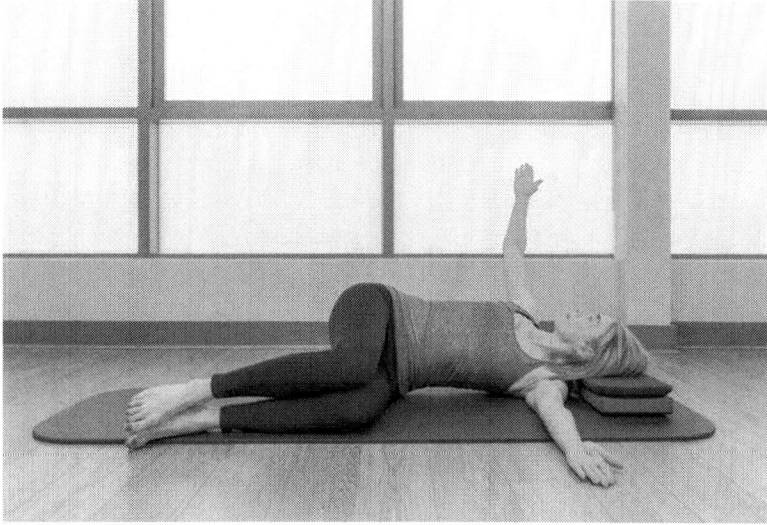

Fig 19

Side-lying challenges our awareness further as we have a narrow part of the body in contact with the mat. This is a comfortable way to enhance rotational movement in the spine. For ideal head and neck alignment, please use a rolled up towel or head cushion to support the head.

Assume a side-lying position with knees bent - as though you were seated on a chair. Place your arms together in front of the body. Establish the sense of heaviness into the points of contact with the floor. Try to maintain a lengthened waist so that the waist is not collapsed into the floor. A useful tool is to place your hand on top of the pelvic half and roll the pelvis forward and back on its side (just like in Exercise 1 and 6). You will feel the waist sink into the mat and then lift up off the mat. Find the middle ground where the pelvis feels comfortable and not fixed in place.

As you exhale, feel the weight of the top shoulder blade drawing down to your mid back. As with the Supine Arm Rolls in Exercise 2, can you get a sense of the upper arm bone being heavier than the forearm, so that the upper arm is able to roll down into the shoulder socket, enabling it to then roll up until the finger tips point at the ceiling? Keep looking at the hand as your neck allows. Do not strain the neck to see the arm.

Once the fingertips are pointing up at the ceiling, take a further exhale and begin to roll the ribs away from the knees - rotating the spine and maintaining the gaze on the hand. Try to keep the arm still and settled in the shoulder socket. Feel the weight of the legs and the other arm resting on the floor. Do not let the moving arm fall the floor behind you - keep it connected into the back of the body. Tip: if you cannot see the inside length of your arm, you have gone too far.

Inhale into the top ribs and feel the ribcage expand. Exhale, holding the position to see if that facilitates any further rotation of the spine.

When you are ready to return, use the exhale to roll the ribs, carrying the arm in its socket back to face the front. Allow the arm to float back down and rest on top.

Repeat 5 times on each side. You may notice one side of the body feels different to the other.

MindBody Connection Moment: Can you keep awareness of the arm moving in space and still connected deep in the body? Can you connect to the rotational power of the spine to bring you back from your arm roll?

9)   Side lying leg roll

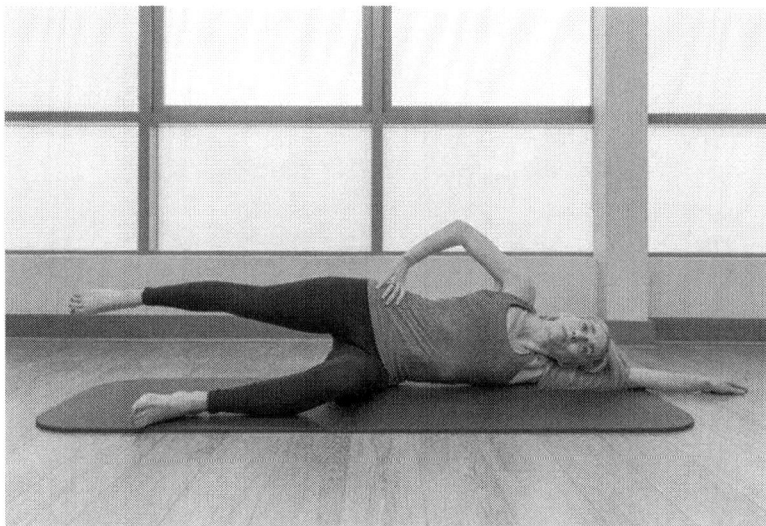

Fig 20

Assume a side-lying position and the resting position of the pelvis as from Exercise 8. You can use a towel or cushion to support your head in this alignment.

Begin with the legs bent as though you were seated on a chair. Then, extend the top leg out until it is straight and in line with the body. It should be as though you were standing on one leg upright.

The aim here is to be able to facilitate a rolling motion of the top leg forward and backwards of the midline without the spine being disturbed. Begin to roll the leg forwards as you inhale - relate the motion back to the supine knee roll and how the thigh bone has the ability to roll and sink into the hip socket. It is the same feeling of the thigh bone articulating in the pelvis, but the challenge is greater because the leg is now long and we are on our side. As the leg swings forward, we aim not to flex the spine or arch the back.

As you exhale, roll the thigh bone backwards until the hip is extended but the back is not arched. There will be a response from the lumbar spine, but it should not overextend.

Notice the rolling action of the thigh bone forward and backwards. Think of the alignment of the leg so that the leg is parallel to the floor and the foot is not dropping down towards the floor. Try to keep the leg at hip height the whole journey forward and back. Keep sending the breath down the leg to continuously create space and freedom in the joints.

Repeat 8 times on each side. Does one side feel different than the other?

MindBody Connection Moment: Do you find greater stability when you allow the body weight to drop down into the side on the floor? Does your leg have greater freedom the heavier the body becomes? How does the breath help facilitate that?

10) Standing side roll

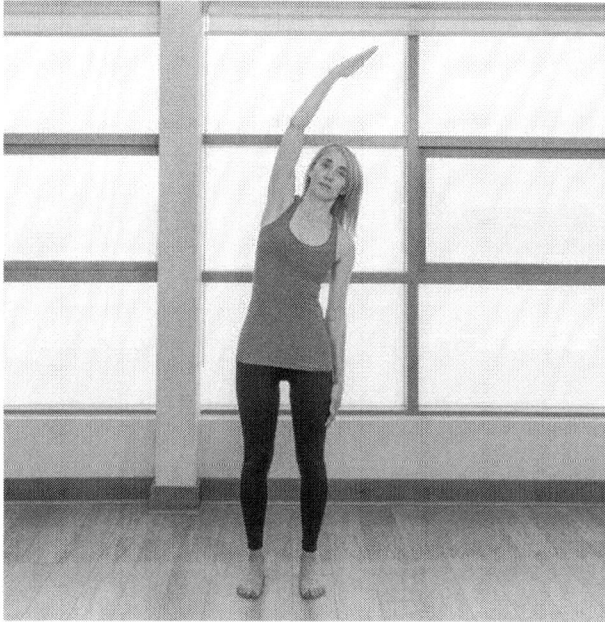

Fig 21

From side-lying challenging our stability, we come to our first standing exercise. This is where the knowledge and awareness gained from the early chapters in the book are really going to be essential. If we are grounded into our feet, conscious of the downward pull of the pelvis coupled with the lightness of the spine, we will achieve greater ease of movement.

Establish a comfortable standing posture - refer back to the early exercises if you need to such as Find Your Sole in Chapter 2. Once you feel connected into the floor, allow the arm to float up and out to the side of the body. Can you utilise the previous knowledge gained in Supine Arm Rolls and Side-Lying Arm Rolls to bring the arm up above the head? The upper arm bone gains a weightier feel than the lower arm so that the head of the arm bone falls and rolls in the shoulder socket. The collarbones remain open and wide.

Continue your arm movement into a spinal movement to the side, feeling the weight shift more to the foot you are bending over.   There is no need to over reach the arm - simply continue the movement into a flowing spinal movement. Let the arm rest in the shoulder socket. The arms are embedded deep into the body - can you allow your whole side body to respond to the movement, rather than just the arm? Does the pelvis stay resting on top of the thighs or do you allow it to shift to help you balance? Try to keep centred.
When you have flexed to the side, take an inhale and allow the open ribcage to expand.

To come back, use your exhale to transfer the weight down into the opposite foot, so that you are drawn back to your centre. The balance between the feet is re-established equally. Use the whole side body to return rather than pulling with your lumbar spine.

Repeat 5 times on each side.

MindBody Connection Moment: As you exhale as you bend and return, can you use the breath to facilitate freedom? Allow the tissue to expand as you bend and contract drawing you back to your centre.

11) Standing Roll Forward

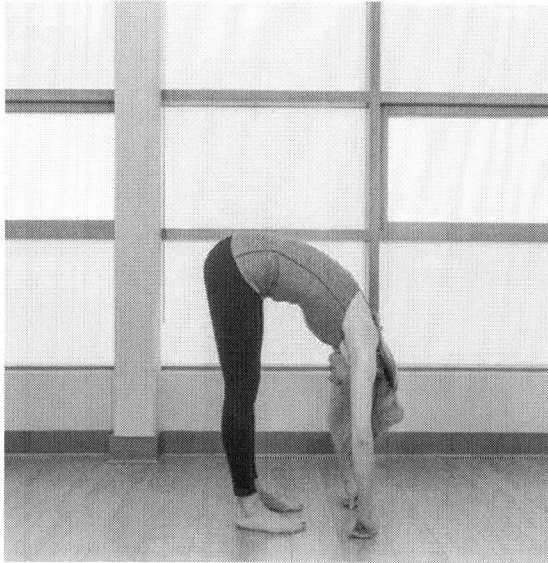

Fig 22

Establish a standing posture with equal balance between the feet. Find your feet and allow them to spread into the floor. This exercise can be practised against a wall too to begin with - the pelvis stays supported against a wall while you roll down.

Feel you are drawn down by the weight of your legs. As the legs get heavier, allow the head to nod and begin to slowly roll forward through the spine on an exhale. We are aiming not to collapse into the joints and hang off the hip joints. Try to find the spine lifting up and out of the pelvis into the roll forward. The spine will lengthen away from the heavy draw of the legs.

As we flex the spine forward and down, notice the abdominal wall draws backwards towards the spine. Ideally we keep the weight balanced through both feet without hinging onto the heels. Take as many breaths as you need to go down.

Allow the knees to bend if you need to on the way down.

Inhale at the bottom and send the breath up into the back of the lungs.

As you exhale, stand down into your feet. Feel the feet dropping down into the floor. Notice the response again of the abdominal wall as it draws up and back into the body. Follow that motion of drawing up and back as you roll back upright re-establishing a standing posture. Can you go down to come up? Tip: your legs should be working as your roll up, allowing the spine to unravel freely.

Repeat 5 times.

MindBody Connection Moment: Can you use your breath to connect deeper into the body? Notice how the breath draws the abdominal wall back in a natural way when flexing the spine. Every time you exhale on the way down explore how the abdominal muscles respond.

12) Standing Hip Softener

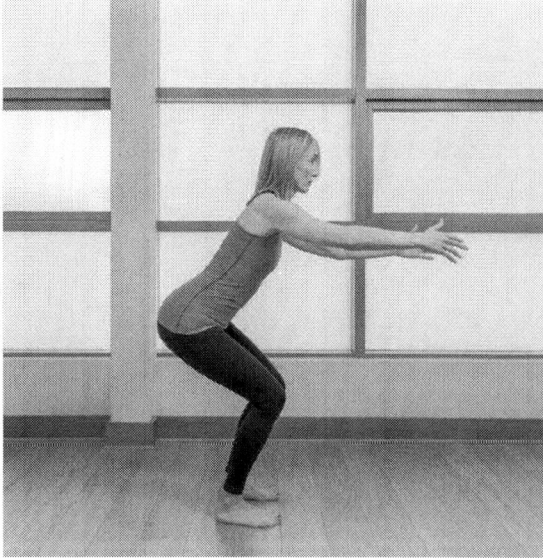

Fig 23

Establish your standing posture as previously discussed. Avoid extreme knee flexion if you experience knee pain. This should feel comfortable throughout the body. Aim to keep the spine lengthened, breastbone moving away from the pelvis.

Rather than approaching this as a squat and pressing down into the joints, allow the hips to soften backwards, which causes the knees to fall forward. The movement is initiated at the hip joint - as though you were about to sit on a chair. As you soften backwards, the arms can float forwards with the shoulders resting on the ribcage. Try to establish a sense of widening of the sitting bones and the front of the hips simultaneously.

Keep awareness of the feet. As we come into our Hip Softener position, the feet are going to need to spread out more into the floor. Soften the feet.

To stand up, rather than pulling yourself up using your spinal muscles, send the feet down into the ground. Again, can you go down to go up? As the legs work more, the spine finds a lightness and lengthens back up into standing.

Repeat 8 times.

MindBody Connection Moment: Can the legs lift you up? Could you stay in this position for a number of breaths allowing the body to simply settle? Try it.

13) Ski feet

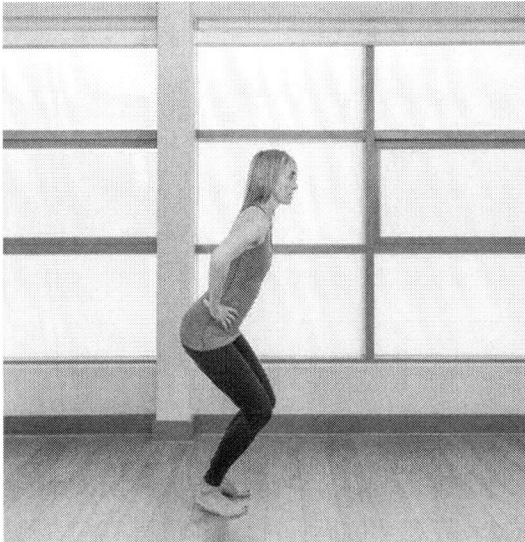

Fig 24

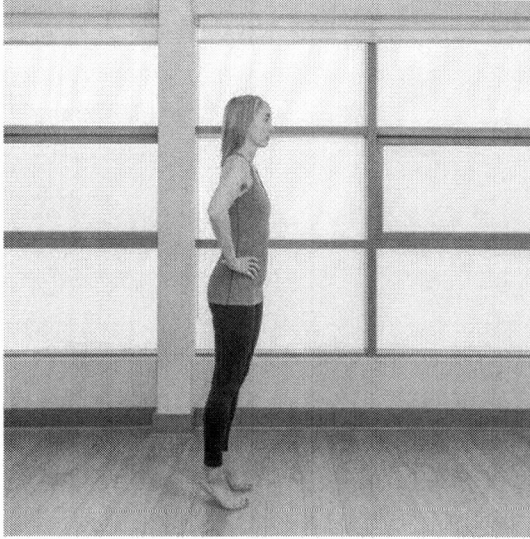

Fig 25

I have named this ski feet mainly because I used it a great deal when working with skiers pre-season. It is a great strength and mobility exercise for the feet, coupled with balance and joint control.

Begin in your standing posture. Allow the heels to rise off the floor so that the weight is falling through the metatarsal heads - big toe and little toe ball of foot. Try to go straight up rather than forward and up.

Allow the hips to soften and carry out the hip softening exercise so that you are in a squat position.

Lower the heels gently to the floor. Stand by sending the weight down into the feet and allowing the knees to open.

Repeat 6 times and then try the reverse of this pattern. You begin in the Hip Softening position followed by a lift of the heels. From this position send the weight down into the balls of the feet to stand up. Finish by lowering the heels slowly back down to the floor.

MindBody Connection Moment: How does this breath change when we feel challenged and unstable on our feet? Can you use the breath to settle the body despite having less contact with the floor?

14) Standing Hip Roll

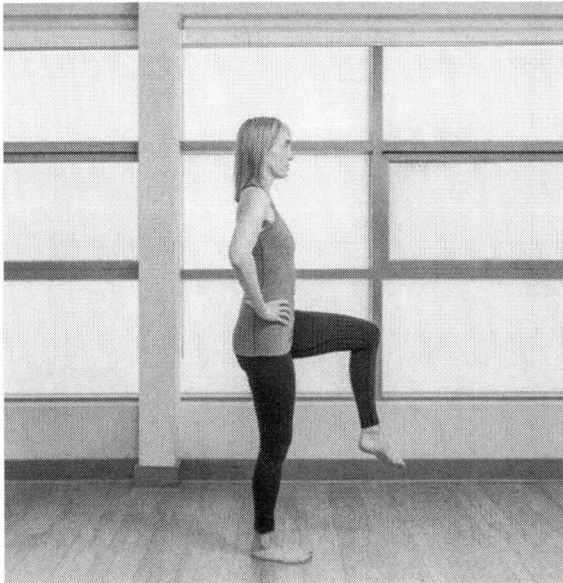

Fig 26

Being upright is becoming more functional - this is where we spend our time. The Standing Hip roll is extremely important - how many times a day do you flex your hip and knee? Climbing stairs, for example.

The Standing Hip Roll has all the same principles as the Supine Hip Roll, but we have less contact with the floor, we are working against gravity and will probably feel unstable standing on one leg.

Before attempting this exercise you will need to be well-established on your feet. You can hold on to a chair if you have any balance disorders.

Assume a standing posture and feel the legs being drawn down into the ground. As you exhale, allow one leg to become heavier. Focus on the weight of that leg. As that leg becomes heavier, can you allow the other leg to become lighter, so much so that it begins to float up from the floor? Allow the head of the thigh bone to rest in the pelvis - feel the weight of the thigh bone and the lightness of the knee. It is like a pendulum - one end swings down giving lightness to the other end. Can the pelvis remain quiet with this movement? In other words, do you feel the need to arch or round your back? If so, try to establish more weight into your tailbone. Tip: try to keep the standing leg knee joint soft.

Hold the position with an inhale, returning the leg to the floor on the exhale. Aim for a slow, controlled lowering of the leg which then allows the foot to settle back into the floor. As balance is established, we are then in a position to try the other leg with minimum disruption to our posture.

Repeat 8 times on each leg.

MindBody Connection Moment: As you hold the position, can you increase the time spent standing on one leg? Can you find a resting place on one leg through the use of the breath to settle the body?

15) Standing Arm Roll

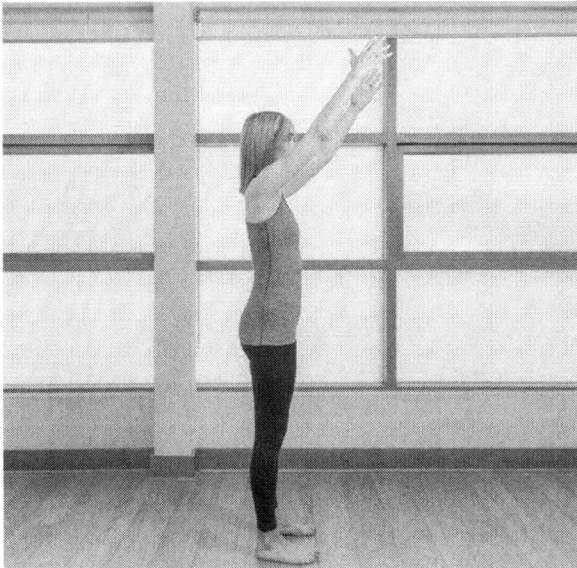

Fig 27

Another extremely important movement that we probably perform dozens of times a day - shoulder flexion - maybe reaching up into a kitchen cupboard to retrieve something. This exercise has the same technical aspect as the Supine Arm Rolls.

Assume a standing posture, feeling grounded through the legs with arms resting by your sides.

Tip: if you have a mirror, stand sideways on to it so that you can see what happens in your spine when you move your arms.

I have deliberately left this one until the end because by now the body will be truly connected and ready to contemplate the action of lifting the arms above your head from the weight of the legs. The arms and the legs are fully integrated together in this movement. As you exhale, allow the feet to widen. As the feet get heavier, can you find a lightness to your arms? Feel the support of the floor. As the arm rises, the upper arm becomes heavier, giving a lightness to the forearm. Feel the upper arm dropping down into the shoulder socket as the arm rises up. The see-saw effect is present - one end becomes heavier whilst the other end becomes lighter. Feel stable in the legs and inhale at the top. Allow the spine to find length from the weight of the legs. The spine will elongate without the binding down of the arms. Feel how the collarbones widen to assist in freeing up the head, neck and shoulders.

On the exhale, feel the arms being drawn back down to the floor by the legs. There is a sense of the arms sliding back into the deep tissue of the torso.

Repeat 8 times.

MindBody Connection Moment: Begin to notice your feet supporting you when you move your arms in daily life.

That completes the selection of foundation exercises. To continue enjoying this programme, head right over to www.pilateswithouttears.com to download your free bonus exercise programme of all 15 exercises.

POST EXERCISE QUESTIONS

- How do you feel after completing your foundation session? Make a mental note of any experiences, new sensations, light bulb moments.
- Were any of the exercises challenging for you?
- How were they challenging?
- Were there any exercises your body resisted?
- Were there exercises you did not want to do? Why was that?
- Which ones were your favourite? Why?
- What did you most enjoy about these exercises?
- What did you discover about yourself on this journey?

The journey does not stop there. We need to build this mentality into our daily tasks and activities. It's so much more than an exercise programme. It is a way of life.

Let's Make it Practical

An important question for you now is how you can apply this new way of thinking and moving to your daily life. It's easier than you think.

The mere fact that you have invested so much time on increasing your body awareness will have made a difference already. Have you noticed a difference in how you stand, for example? Next time you are in the supermarket queue, notice your standing posture. If you catch yourself standing with one knee bent, hip hiking on one side, does a little voice nudge you to move into a more aligned and balanced standing posture? Remember one of our key messages - when we are aware, we can make a change. Otherwise we are blissfully unaware of how our daily habits can affect us. We wonder why we have a tight hip or sore knee after standing at a party for a couple of hours. We may have an idea why now - if we have spent two hours in a hip hiked position. We have disorganised our tent - our tent is happy when all the guide ropes and tensions are in the right place at the right tension. The result of lack of organisation is generally pain, stiffness, aches and niggles of varying degrees.

Initially, until it becomes subconscious, aim to keep scanning your body for clues. Look out for your habits. Standing posture is going to be huge. What about your seated posture at your desk? If you refer to the exercise in Chapter Seven, that will give you a fantastic grounding on how to sit. Try not to slouch at your desk - get some help from your company on ergonomics. Correct screen height, chair height will help in ensuring it is easier to maintain a good posture. Please take regular breaks - sitting is the new smoking! Walk around every hour - move your body!

I wanted to include a point on knee locking because I was a terrible knee locker and I see it a great deal when working with clients. When we lock our knees we are using the knees as stabilisers. The problem is that they are not designed to stabilise the body in standing. It not only puts a great deal of stress and strain on the knee joint itself, leading to wear and tear, but it will also play havoc with your standing posture. If you refer to the standing exercises such as Standing Arm Roll, you will notice that my body is aligned. I have a natural curve in the spine.

Look now at the photograph below - all I have done here is lock my knees.

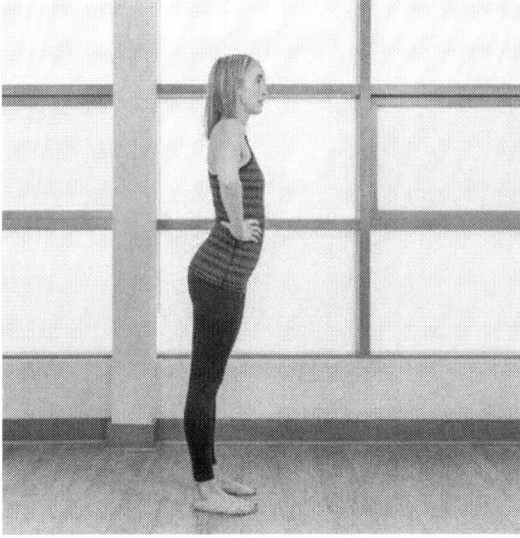

Fig 28

Can you see the effect this action alone has had on my posture compared to the previous photograph? You can see the tension at the back of the knee and the lumbar curve in my spine has increased significantly. Now I used to stand like this but through awareness and working on the softening and noticing when I was holding tension in my body, I was able to retrain my body to hold itself totally differently. If this is how you tend to stand, I am pretty sure you have experienced low back pain or aches after standing for some time. I know I used to as the lumbar spine has been compressed.

When we use our knees to hold us up we block the communication up the chain. It is harder to connect with the feet and use them as they are designed to be used. We now know from Chapter Two how important the feet are in the whole body organisation. So your first homework is to notice if and when you lock your knees.

What about driving - another seated activity most of us have to do to varying degrees. Often a place where we find stress creeping into our shoulders and neck, a forward head position. I recommend to clients to find that weightiness we have talked of in the pelvis. I know it depends on the shape of your car seat - sporty models are going to be a challenge, but try to sit in a peak state. Allow the arms to rest of the wheel, without gripping. The shoulders drape over the ribcage. Think of driving the car from your pelvis so that the arms are free and light.

Pushing a pushchair is an important one - I was one of those new mums with hyper-extended elbows, crushed wrist joints and shoulders up to my ears pushing my baby in his pushchair. I realise now that I was pushing the pram from my shoulder joints and wrists - no wonder I ended up with a chronic shoulder and neck issue! The way I see this now is to try to push the pram from the back of the pelvis. Feel the arms resting on the pelvis so that you can harness the power from the deep waist. This applies just as well to a shopping trolley too.

Most of all, if you get into a stressful situation or while you are performing your exercises, always come back to the breath. I tell my clients, the breath is your thermometer. That is the scale. If you cannot breathe calmly, taking a full breath with ease, something is going wrong. Your breath is the key - it is your very essence. We have seen that simply observing the breath brings mental calmness. It's always there for you and yet it goes unnoticed for most of the day. Use it when you need it. There is a fantastic journey ahead of true mind and body connection with the ability to explore new movement potential and harness greater strength.

Thank you for sharing this special journey with me. I was where you were not so long ago and Pilates literally changed my life. I feel younger now than I did in my twenties and I put that down to Pilates and the mental and physical strength it has given me. I hope you embark on this journey and it brings you the rewards you deserve too.

Further Information

Visit www.pilateswithouttears.com to claim your free bonuses.

The author Jeannie Di Bon is available for one-to-one sessions and Skype sessions. Contact 0044 208 879 9840 or email create@createpilates.com to request further details or to book an initial consultation.

Printed in Great Britain
by Amazon